Celiac Disease Cookbook
for the Newly Diagnosed

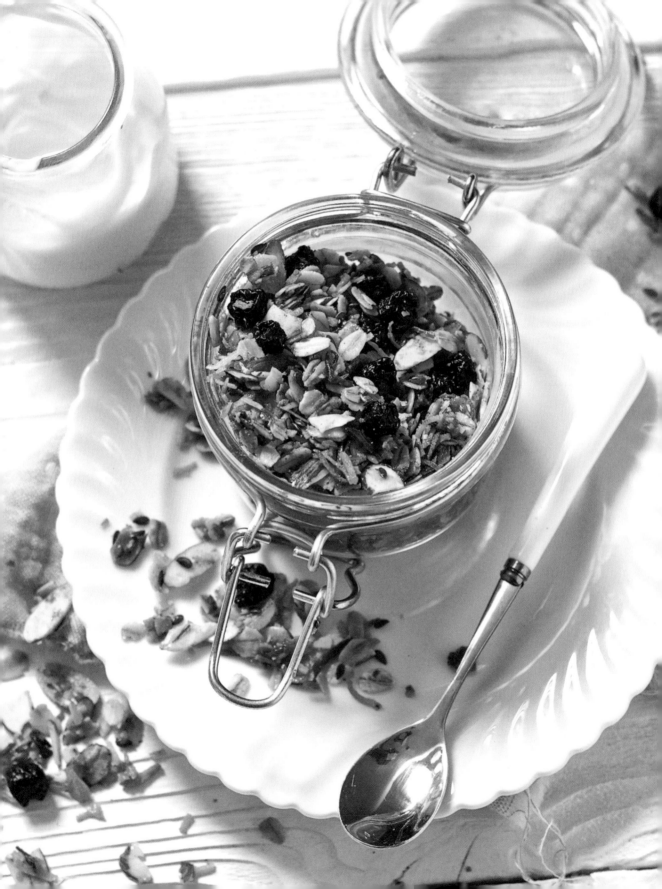

Celiac Disease Cookbook

for the Newly Diagnosed

Guidance and Recipes for an
Easy Transition to the Gluten-Free Diet

Rebecca Toutant, RD, LDN, CDE

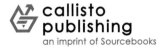

callisto
publishing
an imprint of Sourcebooks

Published by Callisto Publishing LLC C/O Sourcebooks LLC

P.O. Box 4410, Naperville, Illinois 60567-4410

(630) 961-3900

callistopublishing.com

Printed and bound in China

OGP 2

To the women (Mom, Alice, Rhonda, Nina)
who shared with me their wisdom, light,
and love so that I might strengthen others.
And to Grandma Ritger, who showed me
to be fearless in the kitchen because she
so passionately believed "the way to a heart
is through the stomach."

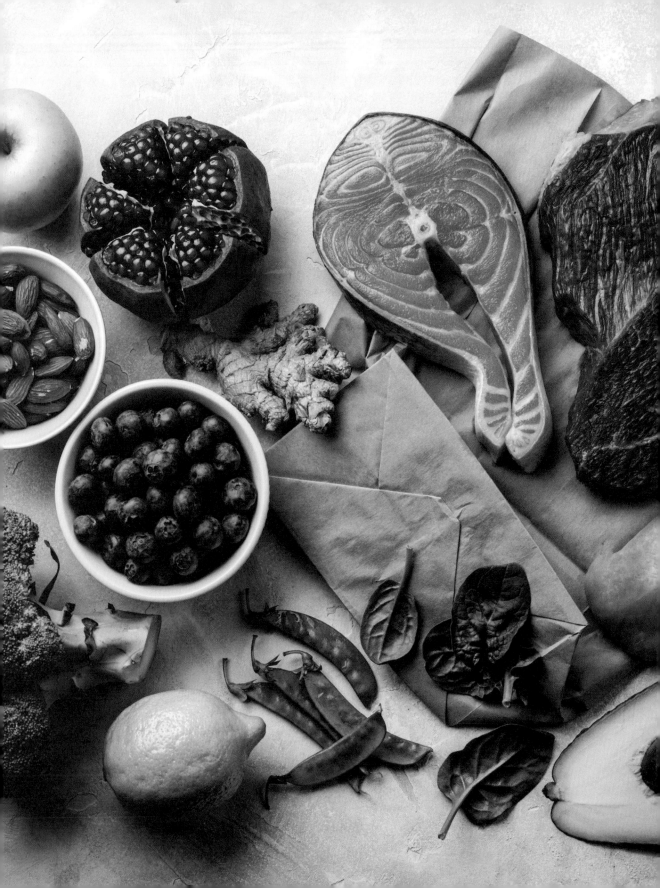

Contents

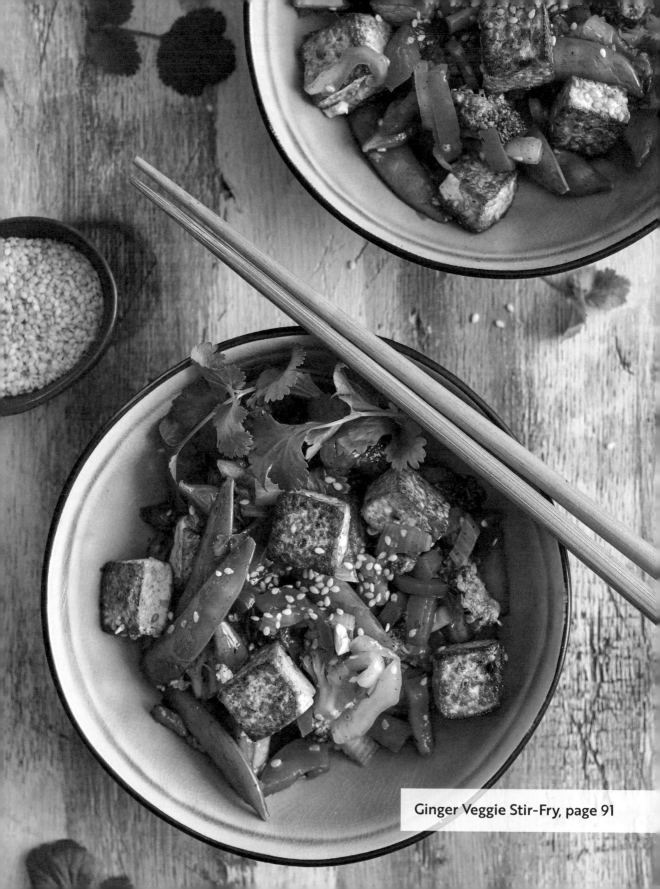

Ginger Veggie Stir-Fry, page 91

Introduction

She walked into my office with a mix of emotions. After years of discomfort, online searches, self-imposed food challenges, and medical tests, she was relieved to have an answer for her stomach issues. Having an answer was a relief but also frightening. She had grown increasingly anxious about food, and she wasn't sure she could live a full-flavored life again. She had already missed out on parties, holidays, and nights with friends due to restrictions and symptoms, but she was ready to get back to it. We spent hours exploring her values and priorities, both in how she wanted to live and eat. From there, we experimented and expanded to find food preparation and eating that worked for the life she wanted. Eventually, she regained her confidence in food and her body.

I've spent countless hours helping people navigate the complex web of food. Many people assume that the answer to health is to limit their food to only what helps their physical body. While physical health is important, doing so at the expense of our emotional needs leads to deprivation. Food is often a reflection of and connection to our core identity and values that stem from our family, friends, culture, and beliefs. It's also a source of joy, celebration, comfort, connection, and entertainment.

Since doing my graduate work on celiac disease in 2009, I've found that the people with the greatest success transitioning to a gluten-free diet were those who didn't let it stop them from living. Following a gluten-free diet doesn't mean giving up every element of joy food brings or locking yourself in the kitchen to prep for the week. Instead, it's about stepping back and getting curious and creative with new ways of assembling old favorites that satisfy your hunger and taste buds, all while evaluating how much time and energy you want to dedicate to food. Celiac disease doesn't define people; it's simply a new approach and consideration in selecting food. There is a learning curve to understand what gluten is and where cross-contamination risks lurk, but once you find your favorite recipes, restaurants, and products, life moves on. To help inspire you, throughout the book you'll encounter Real Talk About Celiac, advice from real people who've successfully and comfortably adjusted to a gluten-free life.

This book focuses on finding creative and compassionate solutions to gluten-free living. Instead of taking away old favorites and the joy of food, it's time to find substitutions and new ways to approach old situations so life continues to feel nourishing.

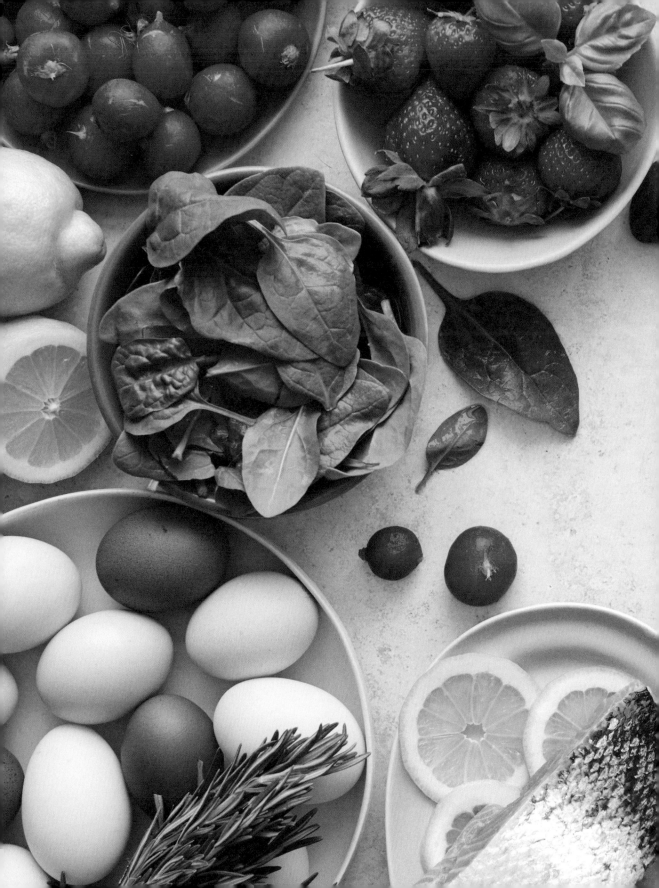

PART ONE

Understanding Your Celiac Diagnosis

A celiac diagnosis comes with a variety of mixed emotions. For the 80 percent of people with celiac disease plagued by symptoms of gastrointestinal (GI) upset, there's relief in having an answer and a "simple" path for relief by following a gluten-free diet. For those 20 percent of diagnosed people with no symptoms, it's not quite clear what the fuss is about or what to do next. Regardless of how someone arrives here, it's important to recognize that there is a growing body of research, solutions, and community around this condition. Rest assured, many people live happy, healthy, and full lives with celiac disease by learning more about how to manage their condition and creating a supportive environment. This book provides a first step in that direction.

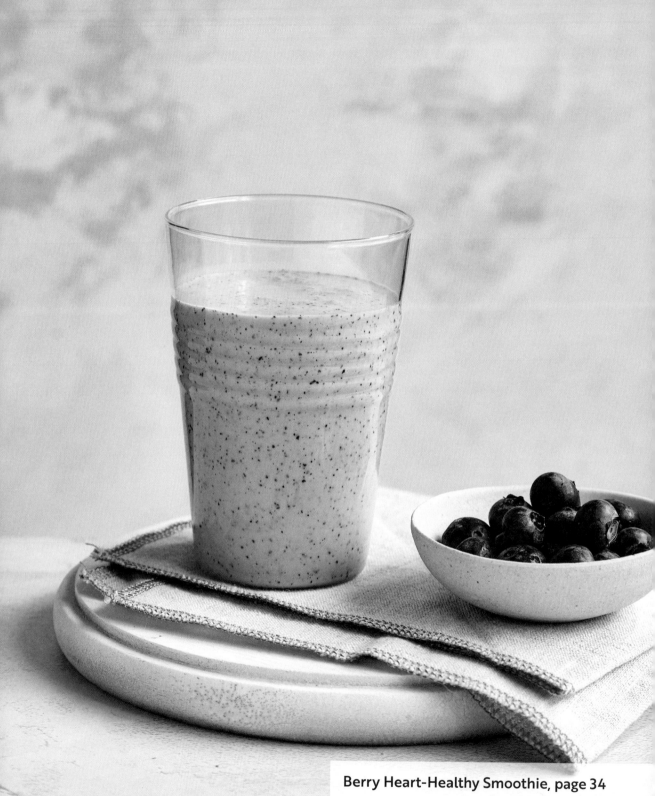

Berry Heart-Healthy Smoothie, page 34

CHAPTER 1

Celiac Disease 101

When trying to orient yourself around a celiac diagnosis, it's helpful to understand what happens to the body when a person with celiac disease comes into contact with gluten. The first chapter of this book explores the basic biology of celiac disease and begins to explore what life looks and feels like when living gluten-free. It outlines where gluten might be lurking at the grocery store, restaurants, and your kitchen, in addition to exploring some of the social challenges to living gluten-free.

What Is Celiac Disease?

Celiac disease is one of the most commonly known autoimmune conditions, affecting 0.5 to 1 percent of the general population. Its prevalence has increased about fivefold since 1975, but it's unclear if the increase is due to improved awareness and subsequent diagnosis or an increase in the disease condition itself. Celiac disease can be genetic and is also more common in those with type 1 diabetes, other autoimmune conditions, and/or Down syndrome. It tends to occur in women more often than men and can be diagnosed at any age—though it's most commonly diagnosed for toddlers and those in their twenties and thirties (likely because other symptoms make it clear something is amiss). However, it's widely believed that the condition is more widespread than what data shows. This may be because the symptoms are easily confused with other conditions, not severe enough for people to recognize as a problem, or absent entirely.

Celiac disease most commonly presents with gastrointestinal (GI) upset such as diarrhea, bloating, constipation, and abdominal pain. It's common to have symptoms similar to irritable bowel syndrome, such as alternating between constipation and diarrhea. Nausea and vomiting may also occur.

Some symptoms and complications of untreated celiac disease come from poor absorption of nutrients. As a result, conditions and effects such as weight loss; anemia; changes in bone mineral density; delayed growth and/or puberty; tooth enamel defects; benign, non-contagious mouth ulcers; and high liver enzymes are common side effects. Many neurological symptoms may also occur, such as headache, paresthesia (tingling of the skin), anxiety, and depression. Celiac disease can also cause changes in reproductive function that may be characterized by late, missed, or absent menstrual cycles; recurrent miscarriages; premature birth; early menopause; and/or changes in the number and mobility of sperm.

Symptoms are triggered when a person with the condition is exposed to gluten, a protein found in grains such as wheat, rye, barley, spelt, and kamut. Exposure can mean ingestion or accidental inhalation. Any gluten getting in your body can result in symptoms, whether that's breathing in flour that's "fluffed" into the air, touching a bagel and then licking your fingers, or even kissing someone who has been drinking or eating something with gluten. (We'll cover ways to mitigate these things in "Go Gluten-Free in Five Steps" on page 20.) In reaction to the exposure, the finger-like projections on the walls of the small intestine, called villi, are flattened and damaged. The intestinal villi play an important role in nutrient absorption. When healthy, they increase the surface area of the small intestine, allowing for appropriate absorption of vitamins and minerals. But when flattened and damaged, nutrients are unable to make their way from the intestine to the cellular structures where they belong. This results in GI upset and malnutrition. Continuous exposure to gluten causes damage to the small intestine, which in turn can lead to malabsorption of nutrients.

For someone with celiac disease, continued exposure to gluten can lead to many acute and chronic health conditions. Issues related to malabsorption of nutrients such as anemia, bone loss, and vitamin and mineral deficiencies are common. Additionally, issues can arise with the pancreas, gall bladder, and central and peripheral nervous system (muscle spasms, seizures, migraines, decreased strength, and loss of feeling in hands or feet). Finally, more serious medical conditions such as infertility and miscarriage, intestinal lymphomas and other GI cancers, dementia, and other cognitive loss are also associated with chronic gluten exposure.

The list of potential health problems from having gluten is frightening, but most long-term complications can be avoided by following a strict gluten-free diet (GFD). That means avoiding all foods, beverages, and medications with gluten and gluten-containing ingredients. With avoidance and time, the villi return to normal and nutrients are absorbed as intended. Villi are regenerated approximately every three days, so long as they are not exposed to gluten. Most people find their symptoms improve dramatically within two weeks, but it can take weeks or months for the entire body to completely recover.

While the treatment sounds simple, it is complicated by the fact that even small exposures the size of a crumb can cause the villi to flatten, even if the person has no physical symptoms. You can be exposed by mouth or by breathing it in, although physical skin contact won't cause a reaction. Once gluten is ingested, there's no way to "undo" the exposure. It just takes time for the body to heal.

Many people live happy, healthy lives while still doing their best to avoid gluten. Fear of exposure cannot and should not prevent one from living. While it's important to try to not intentionally eat gluten, recognize that exposures will likely happen despite best efforts—it's part of living and learning. If exposure does occur, try to learn from the situation and see if anything can be done differently next time.

How Is It Treated?

The only treatment at the time of this writing is strict avoidance of all foods, beverages, and medications that contain gluten. (Even some cosmetics have gluten in them and they should be avoided, too.) It requires a watchful eye and many questions to understand what, how, and where food is prepared. Chapter 2 explores what it takes to create a gluten-free home environment.

Living gluten-free is not as simple as "eat a smaller serving of bread," "eat the meat, not the bun," or "just remove the croutons from the salad." While the amount of gluten matters (more gluten leads to more damage), even a crumb of gluten left over from a misplaced crouton or lingering on a toaster coil can cause an internal reaction, even if the person doesn't have physical symptoms. In this sense, it makes celiac disease more challenging than a food allergy.

For example, with a peanut allergy, a person knows when they've been exposed and can take a medication to reverse the reaction. However, with celiac disease, exposures can occur without a symptom. While celiac won't cause a restricted airway, the only treatment for a gluten exposure is time and future avoidance. No amount of water or laxatives will undo the impact on your body.

There is hope in future medications that may block or reduce the severity of a person's reaction to gluten exposure. However, at present, there is no way for a person with celiac disease to consume gluten and reverse or reduce a reaction. Instead, it's about managing the side effects.

Overcoming Stigmas About Celiac Disease

The gluten-free diet has become more mainstream in recent years due to popular diets and mass media. The benefit of increased awareness is that demand for gluten-free products and labeling has made it easier to navigate the food world than ever before. The downside is that many people aren't aware of celiac disease and why it necessitates a gluten-free diet. Instead, they mistake being gluten-free as a "choice" or "personal preference," like other popular diets. As a result, people don't approach food preparation with the necessary considerations. Because exposure doesn't result in immediate, life-threatening, visible reactions such as those that occur in food allergies, they don't have any evidence of the damage it causes.

This can feel isolating and frustrating for someone with celiac disease. At times, it may feel like one has to prove the existence of illness to validate a request. Some people report difficulty advocating for their needs, such as when asking for food to be re-prepared at restaurants or requesting certain modifications. Advocating and vocalizing needs are the only way to educate others *and* ensure a safe meal. Engaging in a celiac support group either online or in person can help people find comfort, security, and reinforcement.

When communicating your needs with the world, not everyone needs to know every detail of the condition. At a public event with food, where interactions are more short-term, it may be helpful to keep the details simple and say "No, thank you." Some people follow with "I cannot eat that," while others call it "an allergy to wheat" rather than go into detail about the difference between an allergy or defining gluten. Because food preferences and beliefs are popular topics of conversation, be prepared that once you begin to share your dietary needs, curious people will likely push further, share their own knowledge and beliefs, and the conversation will continue. If you'd prefer not to talk about gluten all night, politely declining a dish will end the conversation.

For longer relationships, such as with family and friends, it may feel more comfortable to go into some detail about the importance of the gluten-free diet. It can feel overwhelming to teach people detailed ingredient lists. Instead, consider slowly sharing easy gluten-free recipes and substitutions, such as those in this book. Similarly, always bringing a gluten-free dish to the party not only ensures a safe option but also brings others in on the change. People share food as a way to share a piece of themselves, and that doesn't change with celiac disease. Most people want to support others but need the education and details to make it happen. Remember, you live with your health condition at every meal, every day. Others are just visitors in the experience.

The Basics of a Gluten-Free Diet

Gluten is a protein found in grains such as wheat, rye, and barley. Gluten does not cause harm to the general population. It's only harmful in celiac disease because it triggers an autoimmune reaction. Some people may be confused about this, but consider other food-related conditions such as a peanut allergy. Peanuts are not harmful to most people, but for those with a peanut allergy, being exposed to the peanut protein causes the body to react. There's nothing wrong with the peanut itself; in other words, it's not innately toxic. It's just that some people's bodies cannot handle it.

Gluten has many positive properties. Gluten acts like an elastic glue and helps food hold its shape instead of crumbling apart. It is what makes bagels chewy and cake soft and spongy. It's also a convenient, low-cost filler and thickener for recipes and medications. With so many uses, gluten is found in many processed and prepared foods, as well as personal products.

There are few to no negative health consequences to avoiding gluten. With proper nutrition education and counseling, it can be a safe diet change for all ages. Going gluten-free itself is not nutritionally superior or inferior to other diets. At one time, the gluten-free diet caused some concern due to lack of nutritional fortification. In the United States, many traditional grain products, such as cereal, are fortified with key nutrients such as iron, thiamin, niacin, riboflavin, and, more recently, folic acid and calcium. However, most people without additional restrictions can get these nutrients from eating a balanced diet including a variety of fruits, vegetables, gluten-free whole grains, and animal- or plant-based protein-rich foods. The risk of nutrient deficiencies and imbalances increases when removing an entire food group from your routine, and this is true when it comes to removing all grains from your diet. It's best to talk with a dietitian to gauge the balance of your diet and your individual risk for deficiency.

WHAT TO AVOID

Wheat, rye, and barley are the most common grains with gluten. Some of these items, such as those on the Surprising Suspects list, may or may not contain gluten. So this is not necessarily a list of complete exclusion, but rather a double- or triple-check one. Products that are typically made with these grains or ingredients derived from them include:

Products

- Beer

- Cream-based sauces, such as cream soups, alfredo sauce, and others are typically made from a roux (combination of flour and butter).

- Foods made with wheat flour, such as bread products (bread, English muffins, breadcrumbs, croutons), baked goods (bagels, muffins, crackers, cookies, cakes, corn bread), cereal, and pasta. Please note it makes no difference if the product was made with "whole wheat" or not. All flour, unless otherwise specified, is made with wheat.

- Malt in various forms, such as malted barley flour, malted milk or milkshakes, malt extract, malt syrup, malt flavoring, or malt vinegar.

Common Gluten-Containing Ingredients

- Barley
- Bran
- Bromated flour
- Bulgur
- Durum
- Einkorn
- Emmer
- Enriched flour
- Farina
- Farro
- Flour
- Graham and graham flour
- Kamut
- Malt and malt vinegar
- Matzo meal
- Phosphated flour
- Rye
- Semolina
- Spelt
- Triticale
- Udon
- Wheat
- Wheat berries
- Wheat germ
- Wheat starch
- White flour

Surprising Suspects

- Brewer's yeast

- Brown rice syrup may be made with barley enzymes.

- Communion wafers

- Corn flakes and rice puffs made with malt extract

- Corn tortillas, corn chips, and corn bread may also be made with wheat.

- Eggs served at restaurants (Sometimes pancake batter is used in the eggs and/or the eggs are prepared in a sauté pan or skillet that hasn't been thoroughly cleaned.)

- Flavored milks may contain malt.

- Gluten-free foods prepared in a bakery that also prepares pastries with gluten, as gluten is often on many surfaces and is easily re-distributed. Allergy-catering bakeries will prepare gluten-free foods in a separate space to prevent cross-contamination.

- Lesser known varieties of wheat, such as wheat starch, wheatberries, durum, emmer, semolina, spelt, farina, farro, graham, kamut, khorasan wheat, and einkorn

- Lickable stickers or stamps

- Lipstick and lip balm

- Meat substitutes, such as veggie burgers, seitan, plant-based bacon, and plant-based sausage

- Medications and supplements made with a wheat-based filler

- Milk substitutes, such as rice milk, may contain barley enzymes.

- Play-Doh

- Potato chips made with malt vinegar or wheat starch

- Pre-seasoned and processed meats may have starch or dextrin made from wheat.

- Some food coloring is made with wheat.

- Soy sauce (though tamari is gluten-free)

- Steamed vegetables prepared in the same water as pasta

- Worcestershire sauce and salad dressings may be made with malt vinegar, soy sauce, and/or flour.
- Yogurt with toppings may contain wheat and malt.

GLUTEN-FREE STAPLES

Remember that gluten is only found in grains like wheat, rye, and barley. There's little to no risk that whole foods—such as fruits, vegetables, meat, seafood, beans, and legumes—will have gluten unless they have been processed in some way. Most dairy products also do not contain gluten. In general, the following are naturally gluten-free:

- All fruits, fresh or frozen, not in sauce
- All meats, fresh or frozen, not pre-seasoned or marinated
- All vegetables, fresh or frozen, not pre-seasoned
- Amaranth
- Arrowroot
- Beans
- Buckwheat
- Cassava
- Champagne
- Chia
- Corn (maize)
- Distilled liquors (bourbon, whiskey, gin, tequila, vodka)
- Flax
- Fresh and frozen seafood, not pre-seasoned or marinated
- Fresh eggs
- Gluten-free grains
- Groats (also known as kasha)
- Hard cider
- Millet
- Most dairy and milk products, such as regular cow's milk, almond milk, soy milk, plain yogurt, and cheese
- Nut flours
- Oats (must be labeled gluten-free)
- Potato
- Quinoa
- Rice
- Sorghum
- Soy
- Tapioca
- Teff
- Unflavored almond or soy milk
- Yucca
- White and red wine

There are also many gluten-free pastas and breads on the market made with rice, beans, tapioca, and so much more. Products change each year as manufacturers perfect their recipes and new options come on the market. Here are a few inside tips about the current market.

The most common complaint about gluten-free pasta is that it gets too soft, but brands such as Barilla (gluten-free), Banza, and Trader Joe's brown rice & quinoa pasta hold up strong.

Real Talk About Celiac

"The first grocery trip was tough on my wallet. It's easy to get caught up on the gluten-free cookies, cakes, brownies, crackers, and bread. But I found that once I refocused on foods like potatoes, rice, vegetables, and fruits, I had more food than I realized. Granted I still had my mac 'n' cheese that I ordered by the case. . . ."

Bread is a more controversial topic. The biggest complaint is that gluten-free bread tends to be more expensive with a drier, crumblier texture. Most people agree that gluten-free bread is best toasted. Udi's, Rudi's, and Glutino brands tend to be the most readily available at most major retailers. Other brands getting closer to the "real thing" are Canyon Bakehouse's Heritage Style Whole-Grain Bread, Schär's Hearty Grain, and Trader Joe's Gluten-Free Whole-Grain Bread.

If you can't find a gluten-free bread you love, wraps are a great backup plan to experiment with. Top brands with a gluten-free option are Mission, Rudi's, BFree, Flatout, and Trader Joe's.

A product that has a gluten-free label will most likely be safe to eat because the FDA enforces this labeling and standard. However, remember that a claim such as "wheat-free" does not necessarily mean "gluten-free." Also, not everything that is gluten-free will have a gluten-free label. Some companies choose not to use the gluten-free label because they don't want to take on the risk or labeling requirements. A quick call to the company will confirm whether or not to be concerned about a favorite product.

Building New Eating Habits

Perhaps the greatest shift in following a gluten-free diet is that eating is less impulsive. Food requires a bit of thought and critical thinking to determine the risk and safety. Food is safest when it's prepared in a gluten-free home with gluten-free ingredients. Chapter 2 will guide you in how to set up that process a bit more. But it's not realistic or expected to prepare every meal at home. To make life easier, anticipate and problem-solve ways to eat when home-cooked meals aren't realistic.

Gluten is fairly engrained in many societies. For many cultures, foods with flour are central, such as pasta and Italy or chapati and India. Life without gluten is different, but it's not empty. Luckily, we live in a world where there are many delicious gluten-free substitutes. The gluten-free substitutes may not taste *exactly* like the original, but products are steadily improving as companies learn more about food chemistry. Like any food product, it can take some trial and error to find the right match for your preferences.

Anticipate and plan to eat three or more times each day. Since life moves fast and food is social, having a few options besides bringing everything from home is important. A little time spent preparing and brainstorming now will make it easier when life gets busy.

First, identify a handful of food establishments (restaurants, grocery stores, convenience stores, etc.) close to school, work, home, and travels that offer gluten-free meals or snacks. If your travels take you out of state, connect with support groups for tips, tricks, and food ideas. Many people bring packaged foods in their suitcase or line up a list of grocery stores close to where they're staying.

Once that list is created, keep it handy when friends, coworkers, or family members casually suggest a meal out. If they want to go somewhere that cannot adequately accommodate a gluten-free diet, there's always the option to bring a meal from a close-by restaurant, bring a dish from home, or eat prior to or after going out. If the restaurant has a rule against bringing in outside entrées, consider stepping aside with the manager to explain the situation. Most will be accommodating as long as others are eating there.

Real Talk About Celiac

"I had to learn a lot more about food preparation than I was naturally interested in, but I quickly learned that just because a dish was gluten-free at one restaurant didn't mean it was gluten-free at another. Understanding the cooking process made it easier to predict and avoid risky situations."

A core part of making the gluten-free lifestyle easier is to get more comfortable cooking, which involves learning and practice. That doesn't have to mean gourmet meals or spending every weekend in the kitchen. Instead, it's learning how to make simple favorites such as Avocado-Tuna Salad (page 53), Shrimp Scampi with Zoodles (page 68), and the 15-Minute Chickpea Skillet (page 99)—or it's simply baking some chicken with a side of rice and a salad for dinner in 20 minutes.

Finding Support

Like many life paths, learning what does and does not work for you takes time and practice. For many, food was "easy" before life with celiac disease. You simply ordered what you wanted from any restaurant that looked good. But if this is the first time in your life that you've had to limit your options, it can feel like a loss. Food is not just a biological decision—humans eat for many emotional and cultural reasons.

Starting a gluten-free diet is also an adjustment for friends and family. They don't live with the condition day in, day out and likely won't have the same skills and knowledge as you. That's why one of the most important steps in this process is to share your knowledge and reinforce your needs so that others can help without accidentally causing harm. For example, support systems may unknowingly make mistakes such as:

- Using the designated gluten-free toaster
- Dipping the knife back in the peanut butter after spreading it on their whole-wheat bread
- Picking the croutons off the premade salad in an effort to help
- Calling potato or corn bread "gluten-free"
- Not remembering to clean up after baking
- Mistakenly believing they can "boil" or "sanitize" gluten away

For a time, it will take extra effort and more questions to help them help you. Until that time, it's sometimes easier to rely on backup plans, such as bringing a gluten-free dish to share or eating before or after events. Online or in-person support groups are great sounding boards for ways to navigate tricky situations such as "food pushers," like Aunt Jane who won't stop pressuring you to eat the pie no matter how many times it's explained to her. Stay strong—it will get better.

It can feel lonely and isolating to not engage with food as easily as you once did. Many without serious physical symptoms admit they're tempted to return to old favorites. But remember this is a medical condition with real and serious complications if not treated with a gluten-free diet. There is no way to reverse the internal reaction once gluten has been ingested.

It's common to feel sad, depressed, or anxious. Engaging with groups on a regular basis will make the transition easier. Joining an online group or listserv will lend insight into delicious gluten-free alternatives, local restaurants, or just provide a safe place to vent about difficult situations.

If it becomes a struggle to stay gluten-free, anxiety levels rise during mealtimes, or it feels impossible to eat without fear, connect with a mental health provider and/or a registered dietitian specializing in celiac disease. Both can help you connect with deeper motivations, find confidence in your path, and help you discover ways to enjoy the experience of eating.

Eating Out

Eating out seems complex when first learning about life with celiac disease. But once it's clear what, where, and how gluten might be lurking, it's possible to research the restaurant and ask questions. Be prepared that not every restaurant has the skills to make it happen, even if they tell you they do.

A simple search online will reveal many gluten-free restaurant options. If possible, guide the group to one of these spots for an easier experience. If that's not an option, be prepared to do some investigating for the safest dishes.

The first step is to explore the menu. If they don't have any items designated as gluten-free (or advertised as such), look for dishes that can easily be made with simple whole ingredients, such as grilled meat, poultry, seafood, and tofu without sauce or breadcrumbs. If possible, call the restaurant ahead of time and ask to speak to the manager or head chef. Then explain the situation and ask questions to gauge their knowledge and ability to accommodate. Some restaurants have special menus that are not public, so it's worth asking if they have a gluten-free menu. If not, ask which items are easiest to make gluten-free. It may be helpful to test their knowledge (and staff knowledge) by asking if they have completed a gluten-free training program or how they prevent cross-contamination. Be on the lookout for answers that are specific.

Once at the restaurant, find a way to connect with the manager or chef and explain that gluten cannot be in the food or it will cause you to become ill. If it feels uncomfortable talking with the team or it's not clear they understand, bring a written tool such as a gluten-free restaurant card. These are available for free (see page 140) from many organizations on the Internet and have a brief explanation of celiac disease and the common ingredients to avoid.

When ordering, consider the following:

Soup, Salads, Appetizers, and Sides

- Be on the lookout for and avoid croutons, wontons, and noodles.

- Practice caution with dressings that may contain wheat, flour, and malt, such as cream-based dressings. If it's unclear, oil and vinegar are typically fine. Some people carry a favorite dressing from home.

- In soups and entrées, cream sauces are likely made with a roux containing flour.

- Fried foods that you might think are gluten-free (such as french fries) may be fried in the same oil as gluten-containing breaded products and, as such, are contaminated.

- It's not uncommon for restaurants to simplify food preparation by steaming the vegetables in the pasta water.

Mains

- Avoid dishes with pasta and baked goods (bread, rolls, wraps, pastries, crust, etc.), unless expressly gluten-free.

- Look for dishes without sauces. Cream-based sauces tend to be made with flour, and Asian flavors tend to use soy sauce. Tomato sauce is typically safe.

- Avoid fried foods because they are usually breaded or dusted with flour. Additionally, otherwise gluten-free foods may be fried in the same oil as gluten-containing breaded products, and as such, are contaminated.

- Choose grilled or baked proteins (chicken, turkey, fish) that have not been breaded.

- Simple sides—such as a baked potato, unflavored steamed rice, and steamed vegetables—are typically great choices (unless steamed in recycled pasta water). Once a vegetable is mashed or sautéed, it's important to explore how it was prepared.

Preparation

- Are surfaces cleaned well between dishes? (For example, are the eggs fried on the skillet right after the pancakes?)

- Are there separate gluten-free prep spaces?

- Is there a dedicated fryer for gluten-free foods?

- Are meats marinated or dusted with flour before they are cooked?

What to Do If You Think You've Ingested Gluten

Despite your best efforts, it's likely that a gluten exposure will happen. For some, this may result in a varying array of symptoms in a few minutes or hours. Once exposure occurs, there's nothing that can be done to undo the process. It may be tempting to drink large amounts of water, take laxatives, or even intentionally vomit. But none of these are effective (or healthy).

It's recognized that the symptoms of exposure are unpleasant, and the anxiety of the experience can be upsetting. But for most people without any other health conditions, it does not typically require a visit to a doctor or emergency room. The one exception is when the reaction is so extreme and/or prolonged that the body becomes dehydrated. If it's unclear whether or not to seek medical care, contact your doctor's office about your individual needs and considerations.

The best treatment is self-compassion. Let the mind and body rest as needed while staying hydrated and properly fueled.

> **Real Talk About Celiac**
>
> "I found Chinese and Thai restaurants tricky, but my friends always wanted to go there. I learned that steamed vegetables with chicken and rice are gluten-free since they don't use a sauce. I started carrying packets of tamari and curry in my bag so the dish had more flavor."

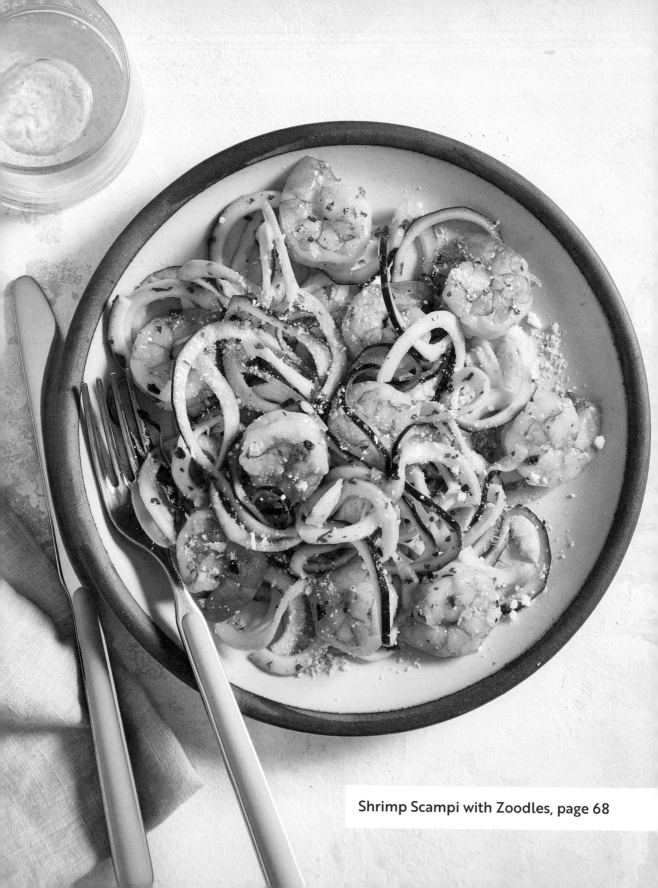

Shrimp Scampi with Zoodles, page 68

CHAPTER 2

Your First 7 Days

Let's dig into your first week of living gluten-free and learn about how to create a solid foundation, starting with your home. Some people live with family, friends, and/or children, and it's important that everyone in the home understands the need for the change and their role in supporting you. For some, that might mean new and separate appliances and cookware. For others, it might be a household transition. Regardless, it's valuable to say goodbye to gluten in the home by deep cleaning the kitchen and reorganizing the pantry to accommodate and restock a clear gluten-free section. Finally, the sample 7-day meal plan in this book will help you get started on your new diet and eating habits.

Go Gluten-Free in Five Steps

Preparation is the key to the gluten-free diet. That means not only making a plan about where and when to eat, but also making your home a safe place. While later chapters of this book focus on cooking, it's important to note that most people do not cook every meal every day. Additionally, not everyone has an interest in cooking. Making your own meals does make the gluten-free diet easier for your health (and your wallet), but it's not required.

No matter your level of interest in food preparation, it's likely that at some point after your diagnosis you'll be in a kitchen, even if it's just to heat up a gluten-free pizza. Understanding where gluten can be found in the home, both inside and outside the kitchen, is an important consideration. Additionally, if you live with other people and they prepare foods with gluten, it's crucial to understand how that can impact you.

Going gluten-free is a big transition that requires planning. These five steps will help get you started on the path to success. Here they are briefly, and then they will be covered in more depth:

1. Get your team (housemates, family, friends, etc.) on board.

2. Remove any gluten-containing foods from the pantry.

3. Clean the kitchen of any potential contaminants.

4. Restock with gluten-free foods.

5. Get cooking!

STEP 1: GET YOUR HOUSEHOLD ON BOARD

Celiac disease affects more than just the person diagnosed. Because food preparation and eating are shared experiences, friends, family, and roommates also need to understand the why and how behind the change. It may come as a shock to some why the peanut butter can no longer be safely shared or why there is a need for two toasters, sponges, and even microwaves.

The first step is to have an honest conversation with those closest to you to explain celiac disease and where gluten can be found. It's particularly important to communicate the issue of cross-contamination, as this is the biggest concern with those living in the same space. It's tough for others to understand how crumbs left over from a sandwich are an issue or that someone you'd like to kiss may need to brush their teeth after ingesting gluten before kissing you again. Be prepared to gently repeat and remind those in the house to clean up and refrain from using designated gluten-free tools. If you share a cooking space, expect to clean before making meals, as well as after. If someone is cooking with flour, it may be best to steer clear of the kitchen for a bit to give airborne particles a chance to settle. Remember, you live with the condition 24/7, while others may only consider it for a moment here and there.

It may be helpful to ask your housemates what type of communication they would prefer. Some ideas are signs on the refrigerator, labels on food and cleaning products, or simple verbal reminders.

If you are the person in charge of cooking for the household, don't feel pressured to make both gluten-containing and gluten-free dishes at every meal. Anyone can follow a gluten-free diet even without the diagnosis. There is little to no risk eating gluten free. Granted, if you're cooking for a family, they may have favorites they're not ready to let go of, but as you'll see in the recipe chapters, there are many delicious favorites that are easily made gluten-free.

As you're communicating with your housemates, these are some food preparation and eating scenarios to consider:

Food storage

- Store gluten-free foods ideally on the top shelf, away from regular bread, pastries, and crumbly foods so that crumbs don't contaminate your food.

- Store foods in plastic tubs or containers, particularly if stored on lower shelves that may be exposed to crumbs.

Food preparation

- Having two toasters is important to avoid cross contamination. Designate one as gluten free.

- Deep clean the microwave (or separate, if it becomes an issue).

- Thoroughly clean all surfaces after baking with gluten-containing flours.

Kitchen cleanup

- Separate towels, sponges, and brushes for cleaning tools with and without gluten.

- Use the dishwasher whenever possible. Rinsing dishes before putting them in the dishwasher can help cut down on potential crumb transfer. It should be fine to wash gluten-touching and gluten-free items together in the dishwasher, especially if rinsed well prior to loading the dishwasher.

- If cleaning dishes in the sink, it is best to wash dishes that have come in contact with gluten separately—separate clean water, separate sponge, separate towel to dry. Otherwise, the sponge and towel can redistribute gluten particles to dishes that have already been cleaned.

- Thoroughly clean pots and pans before and after use.

Real Talk About Celiac

"Having drinks with friends was challenging at first. Bars and restaurants were simple because there were usually hard ciders, pure distilled liquors, and/or wine available. But not everyone has a wide variety at their home. When hanging out at a friend's house, I'd often bring my own gluten-free options and drink responsibly."

Serving

- Provide serving utensils for each dish to make sure they are not used interchangeably.

- Designate and label separate containers for peanut butter, cream cheese, jelly, mustard, butter, and mayonnaise (and other food or condiments that are spread on bread).

- Avoid dipping directly into dips, hummus, salsa, and guacamole with a gluten-containing food (such as crackers, pretzels, or chips).

- Encourage people to put dips on their plate instead of dipping directly into the serving dish.

STEP 2: REVIEW YOUR PANTRY

Now it's time to say goodbye to old gluten faux friends. If it's hard to throw out food, consider donating any sealed goods to a food pantry or taking the items to work for your coworkers. Otherwise, it's time to say adios to all gluten-containing foods, as listed on the Master List of Foods to Avoid (page 138). It's not wise to "use it up until it's gone," as every exposure increases your health risk and prolongs your recovery.

Not all the following items will need to be tossed, but you will need to look at these products' labels to determine whether they contain gluten or clean them thoroughly if the item isn't food. If you live in a household with a mix of gluten-free and gluten-consuming people, you might consider buying gluten-free-designated food preparation items, such as a cutting board or toaster.

Start with the dry goods (cans, boxes, bags). Foods to consider are:

- Cereals
- Breads and pastries
- Fruits in sauce
- Snack foods
- Soup
- Dressing

Then move on to the refrigerator and freezer:

- Flavored yogurts
- Flavored milks and milk substitutes
- Cheese
- Condiments
- Frozen meals
- Fruits in sauce
- Processed meats
- Vegetables in sauce

And lastly, tools used in food preparation:

- Used sponges
- Hand towels
- Wood cutting boards
- Toaster

STEP 3: CLEAN YOUR KITCHEN

If the home wasn't gluten-free before, now is a great time to do a deep clean of any surface that has come in contact with gluten in the past. Any surface exposed to or that touches food that contains gluten should be thoroughly washed and rinsed with warm soap and water.

Toaster This particular tool often has repeated exposure to gluten. Shaking out the crumbs won't solve the problem because the coils themselves touch the bread. With all the internal coils, it may be too much work to clean before and after each use. Instead, most people find it helpful to have a designated gluten-free toaster.

Sponges and towels Sponges are great tools, but they easily collect crumbs and debris. It's best to have a designated sponge that never touches a pot or pan used to make a gluten-containing food or clean up a flour mess. Similarly, towels are an eco-friendly solution for hand and dish drying. They, too, can trap debris, however. Some people find it helpful to color-code. For example, always using green for gluten-free and red for gluten when organizing their cleaning items.

Counters and cutting boards Keep in mind that well-worn cutting boards have more groves that collect grit over the years and are difficult to deep clean. If this is the case, it may be time to get new cutting surfaces and designate them gluten-free. It's particularly challenging if others in the household enjoy baking. As flour is transferred, it's not uncommon for it to become airborne and float around the kitchen, contaminating more surfaces than just the bowl. An air filter can help mitigate airborne gluten. Additionally, you might try requesting that glutenous flour be kept close to the bowl and integrated slowly so that it is less likely to end up in the air.

Utensil and oven drawers It's amazing how many crumbs accumulate in the utensil tray and drawer, as well as in the compartment under the oven. Now is a great time to empty it out and wipe it clean to avoid crumbs getting mixed in with pans and spoons.

Microwave oven When food is microwaved uncovered, it has the risk of splattering around. Trying to prepare a gluten-free food on the same surface risks debris falling into the food in the process. Deep clean the microwave and make sure to protect your gluten-free food by covering it with a plate or paper towel during heating and keeping it on a clean surface.

Pots and pans Tools used to prepare food can be made clean between uses, providing the people you live with do a good job cleaning. If it's cleaned in the dishwasher, it's likely okay to use after, but keep in mind that leftover pasta or crust on a dish may contaminate a gluten-free environment. For this reason, some people find it easier to have a separate set of gluten-free pots and pans.

Table and coffee table Where you eat matters, too. Make sure to wipe down the table, coffee table, or TV trays to avoid accidental exposure. Someone may enjoy pretzels while watching a movie and casually wipe the crumbs away, leaving traces behind. However, those traces can easily be ingested when you sit down and begin to peel your orange. Wiping down spaces before eating on them is an easy way to help prevent this kind of accidental exposure.

STEP 4: GO SHOPPING

Next is the fun part: restocking the kitchen with gluten-free foods! It's helpful to start with exploring preferred meals and create a grocery list from there. Many find it helpful to outline three or four easy breakfast ideas, four or five easy lunch ideas, and four or five easy dinner dishes. From there, creating a grocery list is simple.

Consider breaking the grocery list into sections: produce (fruits and vegetables), refrigerator (dairy, eggs), meat (poultry, meat, fish), frozen (fruits, vegetables), and dry goods (canned and boxed foods). Within that list, here are some tips:

Produce Nothing is off-limits here! Fresh fruits and vegetables are gluten-free. Sweet potatoes and regular potatoes are great starch additions. You'll often find gluten-free meat substitutes, such as tofu and tempeh, in the produce aisle.

Refrigerator In general, plain yogurt, eggs, and regular milk are naturally gluten-free. The only aspects to consider here are any added flavorings to milk or toppings in yogurt that may contain malt or barley.

Meat Chicken, beef, pork, and fish are all naturally gluten-free. If the meat is in a marinade or includes a sauce, be thoughtful about wheat and barley, which may be in the form of starch. Deli meats and processed meats also have the potential for added starches, which serve as a filler and may require some investigation.

Frozen Anything minimally processed, such as frozen fruits and vegetables, likely doesn't have gluten. However, frozen meals can be a bit more complicated. Stick to options that are advertised as gluten-free. You'll likely find prepared gluten-free bread, muffin, waffle, and pastry options in the freezer section or near the gluten-containing bread. Beware of sticker shock. Gluten-free bakery items are often more expensive and have a shorter shelf life than their gluten-containing cousins.

Dry goods Foods in a box, can, or bag will require the most investigation. There are many naturally gluten-free foods, such as rice, quinoa, gluten-free oats, beans, lentils, salsa, and coffee. While it may be tempting to buy items from bulk bins to save on cost, be aware that these items are sometimes cross-contaminated during storage. If possible, it's best to stick with foods that are labeled gluten-free. Once you start digging into boxed foods, it may take a little more time to find truly gluten-free options. Dried herbs and spices are gluten-free. However, if you prefer pre-mixed seasoning packages, make sure to check the ingredient list for any lingering wheat, barley, or malt.

STEP 5: GET COOKING

Now that your kitchen is set up for your success, your housemates are in on the plan, and you've found some foods to try, it's time to get cooking. The next chapters outline a wide variety of gluten-free recipes. Some of the recipes are alternatives to normal gluten-rich dishes, and others have always been and will always be gluten-free. Keep in mind that there's no "right" way to eat a gluten-free diet, but there is a right way for you right here and right now. What works for you now may change in the future and that's okay! Keep trying and experimenting to find the right match.

7-Day Meal Plan

If the new eating process has you feeling overwhelmed, step back and remember that the process of eating has three phases: It's about (1) deciding what to eat, (2) getting the food, and then (3) preparing the food. Here are some tips to make each a bit easier.

Create a plan. Make a short list of your favorite gluten-free foods, as well as simple recipes. Post it on the refrigerator and when indecision strikes, remind yourself that there are many options to consider.

Buy groceries. There are many ways to gather ingredients and keep food handy. Certainly, there's going to the grocery store, but you can also use a grocery delivery service to reduce the effort and have all or some of your needs delivered regularly. They may also have a filter option so that you can search for only gluten-free foods. Many meal delivery services advertise gluten-free recipes as well, which could support some of your meal preparation and expand your recipe library.

Get cooking. How much time and energy do you have to invest in food preparation? Are some days easier than others? Would doing a little meal prep on Sunday make the week ahead easier? Start by outlining which days you have time and energy to cook and which days make the most sense for leftovers or going out to eat. Even having a "theme" assigned to a day can be helpful (e.g., Taco Tuesday or Chicken Wednesday). It gives you a starting block to make meals as easy or complex as you'd like.

The following meal plan is an example of just that. Most people rotate the same one or two breakfast options, and lunch is often leftovers from the previous night or something simple in a pinch. And while some cook a fresh dinner each day, it's more common to do it just a few times a week.

Setting Expectations

Most people begin to experience relief within two weeks of being gluten-free. Others, however, take a bit more time to work through issues around food preparation and cross-contamination. Still others are plagued by GI symptoms due to other chronic conditions, stress, or additional food sensitivities. You may notice your weight increase as nutrients are absorbed and your body is re-nourished. This is natural and normal, and it does not mean you've done something wrong.

Some newly diagnosed people have difficulty digesting lactose, a sugar found in some dairy products. However, once gluten is removed from the diet and the villi heal, they find that they can enjoy lactose-rich foods without a problem. Initially, it may be helpful to avoid high-lactose foods such as cow's milk, and soft or fresh cheeses. But typically Greek yogurt; aged, hard cheese; and butter have little to no lactose. Additionally, gluten-free oats may be an issue for some, particularly early on in the diagnosis. Talk to your doctor about reintroducing gluten-free oats.

Sudden dietary changes can bring some relief, but sometimes they can trigger discomfort. For example, if you didn't eat many vegetables before and now are having a few cups each meal, it takes your body time to adjust. In the interim, you may produce more gas and feel bloated. For most, this side effect goes away with time and continued exposure to high-fiber foods. However, if it does not, it may be worth consulting a qualified health professional to rule out any other food intolerances.

One of the biggest mistakes people make in shifting to the gluten-free diet is taking grains and starches out of the diet completely and trying to rely on only fruits, vegetables, and meats. Grains and starches provide a variety of B vitamins and serve as a rapid source of energy. Entirely removing grains from your diet will likely leave you feeling tired, depleted, hungry, and unsatisfied. Eating too little also tends to leave people ravenous and increases cravings for sweets.

Another mistake people make is buying a large amount of gluten-free convenience foods, such as bread and snacks. Often these foods are more expensive for a smaller portion with a shorter shelf life. Remember there are many naturally gluten-free grains and starches, such as rice, beans, potato, and rice crackers.

Anxiety and stress around trying to be gluten-free is real and can have a legitimate impact on physical and mental health. If you're struggling with fear of food or eating with others, consult with your medical provider immediately. It's not uncommon to spiral into disordered eating after a fear of food diagnosis. Additionally, if you feel overwhelmed and tempted to quit the diet, a registered dietitian can help you create a plan to better ease into the transition. Any step you make is better than none.

THE PLAN

	BREAKFAST	SNACK
MON	Broccoli and Ham Crustless Mini Quiche (page 43) with banana	Apple and almonds
TUES	Oatmeal Cakes with Cinnamon and Fruit (page 47)	Hardboiled eggs and an apple
WED	Yogurt with blueberries and Hearty Spiced Granola (page 42)	Banana with nut butter
THURS	Leftover Broccoli and Ham Crustless Mini Quiche with banana	No-Bake Monster Cookies (page 125)
FRI	Leftover Oatmeal Cakes with Cinnamon and Fruit	Apple and almonds
SAT	Yogurt with blueberries and Hearty Spiced Granola	Hardboiled eggs and an apple
SUN	Belgian-Style Waffles (page 46) with fruit compote	Banana with nut butter

Dessert Ideas: No-Bake Monster Cookies (page 125) or Cookie "Dough" Dip (page 126) with gluten-free graham crackers are two simple ways to satisfy your sweet tooth during the week.

LUNCH	SNACK	DINNER
Avocado-Tuna Salad (page 53) on gluten-free bread with baby carrots	Greek yogurt and ½ cup berries	Chili-Ginger Salmon over Spinach Salad (page 54)
Rainbow Grain Bowl (page 102)	Sun-Dried Tomato-Basil Hummus (page 108) with rice crackers and carrots	15-Minute Chickpea Skillet (page 99)
Leftover 15-Minute Chickpea Skillet	Turkey jerky and apple	Spiced Peach Chicken (page 75)
Leftover Spiced Peach Chicken	Edamame	Honey Pork Tenderloin (page 77)
Savory Tuna Patties (page 70) on gluten-free bread with chips	Roasted Edamame (page 113)	Hearty Mexican-Style Skillet (page 98)
Shrimp Scampi with Zoodles (page 68)	Rice crackers and Sun-Dried Tomato Basil Hummus (page 108) with grapes	Out to eat!
Chicken Vegetable Soup (page 61)	No-Cook Spinach Artichoke Dip (page 109) and chips	Shrimp Scampi with Zoodles (page 68)

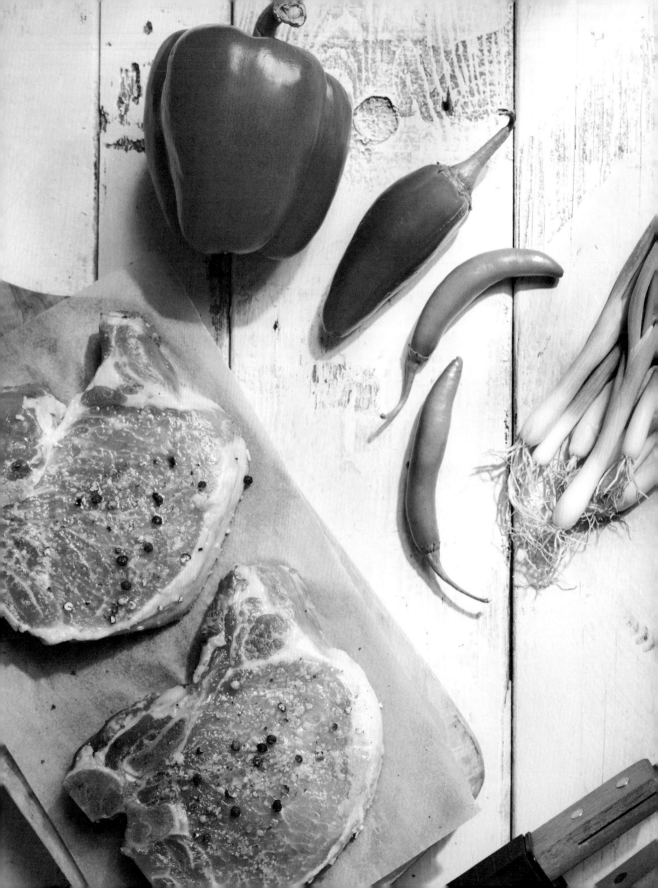

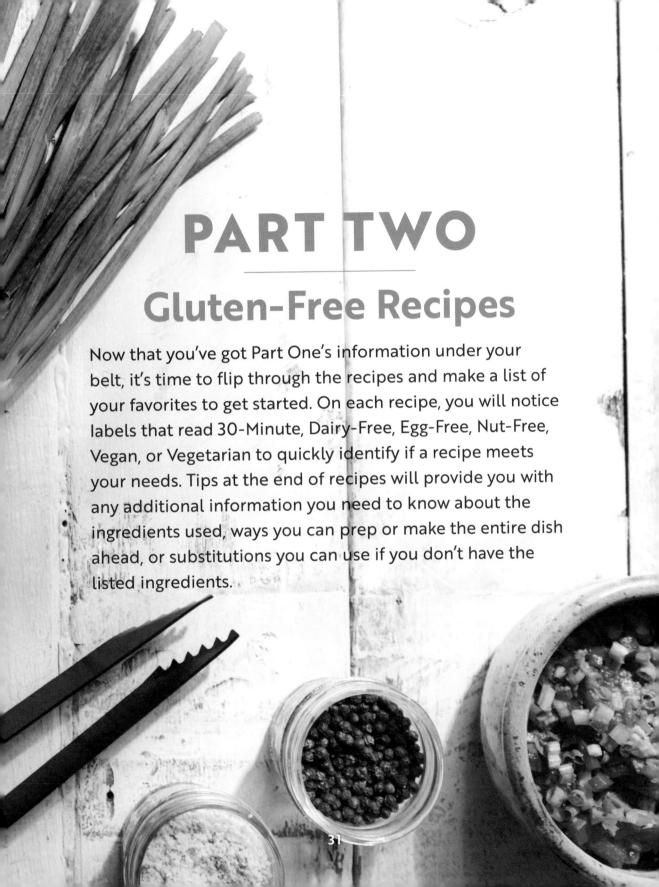

PART TWO

Gluten-Free Recipes

Now that you've got Part One's information under your belt, it's time to flip through the recipes and make a list of your favorites to get started. On each recipe, you will notice labels that read 30-Minute, Dairy-Free, Egg-Free, Nut-Free, Vegan, or Vegetarian to quickly identify if a recipe meets your needs. Tips at the end of recipes will provide you with any additional information you need to know about the ingredients used, ways you can prep or make the entire dish ahead, or substitutions you can use if you don't have the listed ingredients.

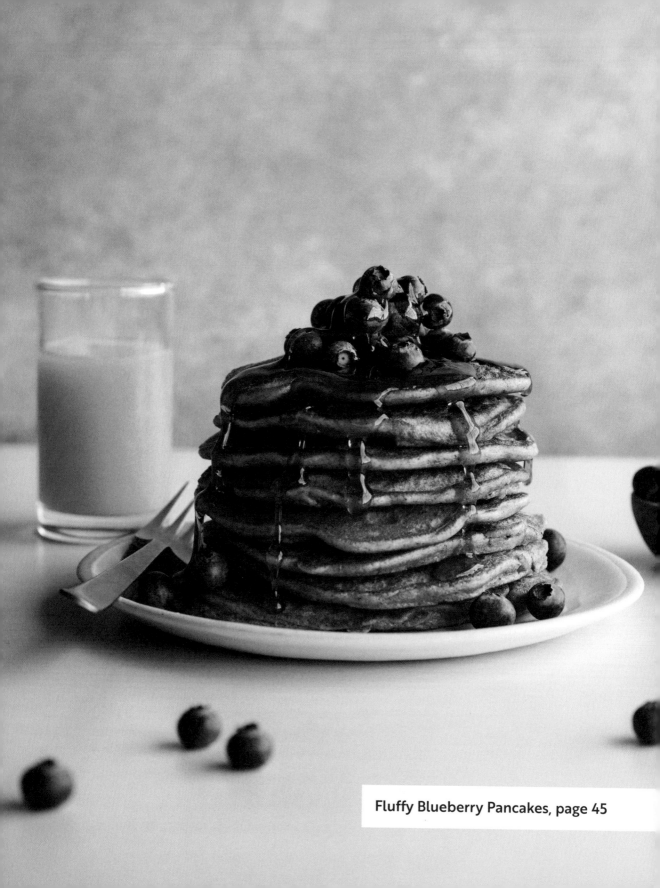

Fluffy Blueberry Pancakes, page 45

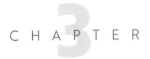

CHAPTER 3

Smoothies and Breakfast

Berry Heart-Healthy Smoothie

Prep time: 5 minutes

A smoothie is only as good as its ingredients. This recipe uses avocado for a dose of heart-healthy fat and satisfaction. For more fiber, consider adding 1 teaspoon ground flaxseed or chia seeds.

2 cups whole milk

1 cup plain or vanilla
  yogurt or kefir

1 cup mixed berries
  (fresh or frozen)

½ avocado

4 ice cubes (if not using
  frozen fruit)

In a blender (or if using an immersion blender, in a large mason jar), combine the milk, yogurt, berries, avocado, and ice (if using) and blend until smooth. If you find the smoothie too thick for your preference, slowly add more water or milk to achieve your desired consistency. Pour into glasses and enjoy!

Per Serving: Calories: 350; Fat: 16g; Saturated Fat: 6g; Carbohydrates: 33g; Fiber: 6g; Sugar: 24g; Protein: 16g; Iron: 1mg; Sodium: 200mg

SERVES 2

30-MINUTE
EGG-FREE
NUT-FREE
VEGETARIAN

Ingredient Tip: Use frozen fruit instead of ice cubes for a thicker smoothie.

Refreshing Green Smoothie

Prep time: 5 minutes

At first glance, this combination of ingredients may surprise you, but it's one of the most refreshing ways to start the day. It provides year-round healing properties as the vitamin C in kiwi and anti-inflammatory properties of ginger help boost the immune system.

1 cucumber, peeled

2 kiwi fruits, peeled

1 cup plain yogurt or kefir

2 tablespoons cilantro leaves

2 teaspoons minced and peeled fresh ginger or ½ teaspoon ground ginger

6 ice cubes

SERVES 2

30-MINUTE

EGG-FREE

NUT-FREE

VEGETARIAN

In a blender (or if using an immersion blender, in a large mason jar), combine the cucumber, kiwi fruits, yogurt, cilantro, ginger, and ice and process until smooth. If you find the smoothie too thick for your preference, slowly add more water or milk of choice to achieve your desired consistency. Pour into glasses and enjoy!

Substitution Tip: For more refreshment and probiotics without the lactose, use ginger-flavored kombucha instead of yogurt or kefir.

Per Serving: Calories: 163; Total Fat: 2g; Saturated Fat: 1g; Carbohydrates: 26g; Fiber: 3g; Sugar: 18g; Protein: 9g; Iron: 1mg; Sodium: 92mg

Banana Spice Smoothie

Prep time: 5 minutes

This smoothie is a fantastic way to ease into a winter morning. The combination of cinnamon and nutmeg lends spice and warmth to the winter season and can help give the immune system a boost.

2 bananas, peeled

2 cups vanilla yogurt or kefir

1 cup whole milk

½ teaspoon vanilla extract

½ teaspoon ground cinnamon

¼ teaspoon ground nutmeg

12 ice cubes

SERVES 2

30-MINUTE
EGG-FREE
NUT-FREE
VEGETARIAN

In a blender (or if using an immersion blender, in a large mason jar), combine the bananas, yogurt, milk, vanilla, cinnamon, nutmeg, and ice and process until smooth. If you find the smoothie too thick for your preference, slowly add more water or milk of choice to achieve your desired consistency. Pour into glasses and enjoy!

Per Serving: Calories: 340; Total Fat: 6g; Saturated Fat: 4g; Carbohydrates: 50g; Fiber: 3g; Sugar: 35g; Protein: 20g; Iron: 1mg; Sodium: 230mg

Substitution Tip: Try a plant-based milk instead of yogurt or kefir for a lactose-free drink. Use frozen bananas instead of ice cubes for a thicker drink. Not a fan of bananas? Use ½ cup canned pumpkin with 1 scoop vanilla protein powder to make it work for you.

Orange Kiss Smoothie

Prep time: 5 minutes

Vegetables in a smoothie scare some people, but you won't notice them here. This smoothie has the taste, color, and energy of a summer day, while boasting a hearty dose of fiber, vitamin C, and vitamin K.

2 cups chopped peaches (fresh or frozen)

1 cup plain yogurt or kefir

2 oranges, peeled, or 1 cup orange juice

½ cup shredded carrot

1 tablespoon minced and peeled fresh ginger or ½ teaspoon ground ginger

In a blender (or if using an immersion blender, in a large mason jar), combine the peaches, yogurt, oranges, carrots, and ginger and process until smooth. If you find the smoothie too thick for your preference, slowly add more water or milk of choice to achieve your desired consistency. Pour into glasses and enjoy!

Per Serving: Calories: 250; Total Fat: 2g; Saturated Fat: 2g; Carbohydrates: 48g; Fiber: 8g; Sugar: 41g; Protein: 10g; Iron: 1mg; Sodium: 106mg

SERVES 2

30-MINUTE
EGG-FREE
NUT-FREE
VEGETARIAN

Substitution Tip: Try your favorite plant-based milk or yogurt for a lactose-free drink. You can also use ginger kombucha instead of ginger and yogurt for an extra boost of probiotics and refreshment.

Satisfying Overnight Oats

Prep time: 5 minutes, plus 3 hours to chill

Overnight oats provide a delicious, convenient no-cooking-required way to start the morning. You can experiment with a variety of ingredient combinations—try adding dried fruit, fresh fruits, nut butter, or yogurt.

1 cup whole milk

½ cup gluten-free oats

½ cup fresh or
frozen blueberries

1 tablespoon nut butter
or 2 tablespoons
crushed nuts or seeds
of choice

1 teaspoon honey, maple
syrup, or brown sugar

SERVES 1

30-MINUTE

EGG-FREE

VEGETARIAN

1. In a mason jar or other container with a lid, combine the milk, oats, blueberries, nut butter, and honey. Cover, shake well, and refrigerate for at least 3 hours or up to 2 days.

2. Stir and enjoy! If you prefer a warm dish, microwave for 1 to 2 minutes.

Per Serving: Calories: 454; Total Fat: 17g; Saturated Fat: 6g; Carbohydrates: 65g; Fiber: 8g; Sugar: 27g; Protein: 17g; Iron: 2mg; Sodium: 355mg

Ingredient Tip: Add 1 teaspoon chia or flaxseeds for a boost of fiber and heart-healthy fats. The addition of your favorite dry fruits like cherries or cranberries adds extra zest and fiber.

Substitution Tip: If you are avoiding oats, you can also use 1 tablespoon chia seeds, 2 tablespoons hemp hearts, and 2 tablespoons coconut flour to create your own gluten-free cereal.

Real Talk About Celiac

"I'm always running late in the morning. Instead of skipping breakfast, I grab a piece of fruit on my way out the door and enjoy with the gluten-free oats that I keep in my desk at work."

Hot Quinoa Cereal with Banana and Peanut Butter

Prep time: 10 minutes / *Cook time:* 20 minutes

Quinoa is a versatile gluten-free grain that's high in protein and fiber. It works well for those who can't tolerate oats and offers a soft, fluffy texture.

1½ cups water or milk

1 cup quinoa, rinsed

½ teaspoon ground cinnamon

¼ teaspoon salt

1 teaspoon maple syrup or honey

Sliced banana, for serving

4 tablespoons peanut butter, for serving

SERVES 4

30-MINUTE

EGG-FREE

Substitution Tip: Replace the banana and peanut butter with ingredients like apples, blueberries, peaches, walnuts, almonds, or cocoa powder.

1. In a saucepan, combine the water, quinoa, cinnamon, and salt. Bring to a boil over medium heat. Reduce the heat to low and cook, covered, until the water is absorbed and the quinoa is tender, 15 to 20 minutes.

2. Remove from the heat and let stand, covered, for 5 minutes. Fluff and divide among bowls, and drizzle with syrup or honey. Serve topped with banana slices and peanut butter.

Per Serving: Calories: 207; Total Fat: 5g; Saturated Fat: 1g; Carbohydrates: 32g; Fiber: 3g; Sugar: 5g; Protein: 9g; Iron: 2mg; Sodium: 193mg

Eggs in a Rainbow Basket

Prep time: 5 minutes / *Cook time:* 5 to 8 minutes

In this recipe, you can put your eggs in one basket. It's a fun, colorful spin on an old classic that will delight kids and adults alike.

1 bell pepper, cut
    into 4 rings

4 large eggs

¼ cup feta cheese

Salt

Freshly ground
    black pepper

SERVES 4

30-MINUTE

NUT-FREE

VEGETARIAN

1. Heat a nonstick sauté pan or skillet over medium heat. Place the bell pepper rings in the hot skillet and crack the eggs into the bell pepper rings. Cook for 2 to 3 minutes, until the bottom holds together, and the corners are browned.

2. Gently flip and cook for 2 to 3 more minutes, until desired doneness is reached.

3. Sprinkle feta over top. Season with salt and pepper.

Substitution Tip: Use egg whites or egg substitute to reduce the saturated fat and cholesterol. For a fun flair, add your favorite herbs and spices, such as chives, garlic, or curry.

Per Serving: Calories: 74; Total Fat: 5g; Saturated Fat: 2g; Carbohydrates: 1g; Fiber: 1g; Sugar: 2g; Protein: 7g; Iron: 1mg; Sodium: 225mg

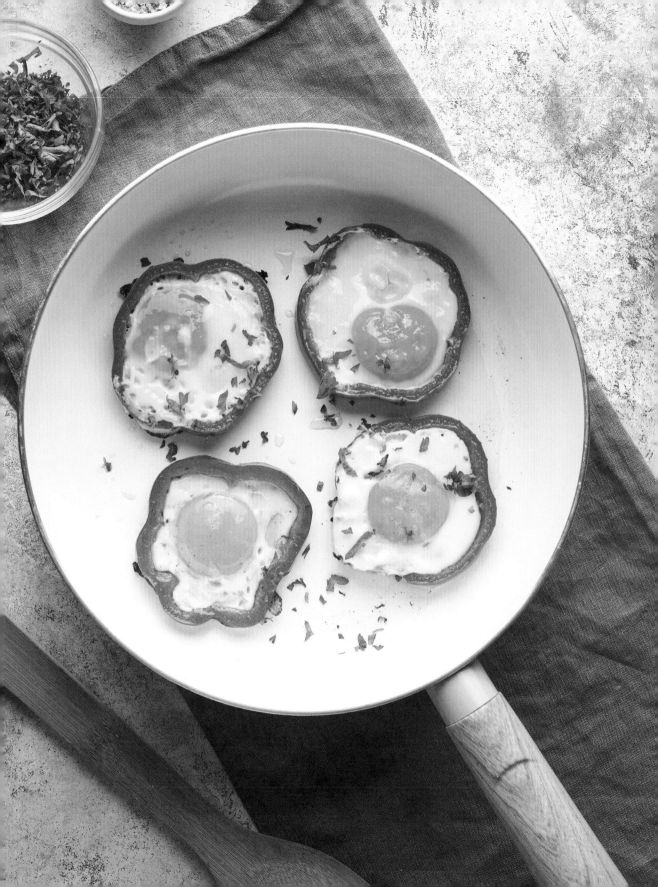

Hearty Spiced Granola

Prep time: 10 minutes / *Cook time:* 20 minutes

Homemade granola adds a delicious crunch to yogurt, cottage cheese, oatmeal, or just plain old cereal. Making it at home not only keeps it gluten-free but also makes your home smell divine. To make this oat-free, increase the amount of nuts and seeds to 3 cups. Experiment with different nuts and seeds, such as almonds, walnuts, or sunflower seeds, and dried fruits, such as dates, apricots, cranberries, or cherries.

4 cups gluten-free
   rolled oats

1 cup nuts or seeds

¼ cup vegetable oil or
   coconut oil

¼ cup honey

1 tablespoon
   ground cinnamon

1 teaspoon
   vanilla extract

½ teaspoon
   ground nutmeg

Dash salt

½ cup dried fruit

SERVES 12

**30-MINUTE
DAIRY-FREE
VEGETARIAN**

Ingredient Tip: Add 2 tablespoons whole flaxseed or chia seeds after cooking for a boost of fiber and heart-healthy fat.

Storage Tip: Store in an airtight container for 2 weeks. If you prefer your dry fruit on the softer side, add it at the time of serving instead of storing it with the granola mixture.

1. Preheat the oven to 325°F. Line a baking sheet with parchment paper.

2. In a large bowl, combine the oats, nuts, vegetable oil, honey, cinnamon, vanilla, nutmeg, and salt.

3. Pour mixture onto the prepared baking sheet and bake, stirring every 5 minutes, for 15 to 20 minutes, until golden.

4. Remove and let cool. Mix in the dried fruit.

Per Serving: Calories: 275; Total Fat: 12g; Saturated Fat: 2g; Carbohydrates: 37g; Fiber: 5g; Sugar: 12g; Protein: 7g; Iron: 2mg; Sodium: 100mg

Broccoli and Ham Crustless Mini Quiche

Prep time: 10 minutes / *Cook time:* 25 minutes

A crustless mini quiche makes a delicious, protein-rich start to your morning. This egg-based dish can be made with a variety of fresh vegetables (such as bell peppers, broccoli, or cauliflower) and proteins (such as ham, bacon, turkey, or chicken). Baked egg can be tough to clean (even on a well-greased pan), so use parchment muffin papers or reusable muffin liners to make cleanup easy.

12 large eggs

½ cup whole milk or cream

½ cup water

¼ teaspoon salt

¼ teaspoon freshly ground black pepper

¼ teaspoon garlic powder

1 cup finely chopped broccoli florets

1 cup dairy-free shredded sharp cheddar cheese, divided

¼ cup chopped onion

½ cup cooked and diced ham

SERVES 8

NUT-FREE

Substitution Tip:
This recipe calls for dairy-free cheese, which can be helpful in the initial weeks of recovery. If lactose is not a problem, use your cheese of choice, such as Swiss or sharp cheddar.

Per Serving: Calories: 143; Total Fat: 9g; Saturated Fat: 3g; Carbohydrates: 5g; Fiber: 1g; Sugar: 2g; Protein: 9g; Iron: 1mg; Sodium: 310mg

1. Preheat the oven to 375°F. Line 8 cups of a muffin tin with muffin liners.

2. In a large bowl, whisk the eggs, milk, water, salt, pepper, and garlic powder together. Mix in the broccoli, ½ cup of cheese, onion, and ham.

3. Scoop the mixture into the muffin cups, leaving ¼ inch from the top.

4. Sprinkle the remaining ½ cup of cheese over the tops.

5. Bake for 20 to 25 minutes, until the quiches are firm and the cheese is slightly golden.

6. Let cool 5 to 10 minutes before removing. Let cool completely before storing in an airtight container in the refrigerator for up to 5 days or freezer up to 2 weeks.

Ham and Cheese Breakfast Casserole

Prep time: 15 minutes / *Cook time:* 50 minutes

On days when you want a satisfying breakfast or are hosting for a holiday, a breakfast casserole is a great way to entertain. It's simple to assemble and no monitoring is necessary—just prep, bake, and walk away.

3 cups frozen
   hash browns

1 cup chopped
   ham, divided

12 large eggs

1 cup whole milk

2 cups shredded
   sharp cheddar
   cheese, divided

1 bell pepper, chopped

½ cup chopped onion

1 teaspoon garlic powder

SERVES 10

NUT-FREE

Make Ahead Tip: Prep this dish the night before for an easy entertaining breakfast option.

Substitution Tip: Like a quiche, this dish can be made with a variety of vegetables and meat options. If you want to lighten up the sodium and saturated fat, use Swiss cheese instead of cheddar.

1. Preheat the oven to 350°F. Grease a 9-by-13-inch baking dish.

2. Place the frozen hash browns in the baking dish and layer ½ cup of ham over the top.

3. In a large bowl, whisk the eggs and milk. Stir in 1 cup of cheese, the bell pepper, onion, and garlic powder. Pour the mixture over the potatoes and ham.

4. Bake for 25 minutes. Carefully remove from the oven and sprinkle the remaining ½ cup of ham and remaining 1 cup of cheese over the top. Bake for an additional 20 to 30 minutes, until golden brown.

Per Serving: Calories: 417; Total Fat: 14g; Saturated Fat: 7g; Carbohydrates: 48g; Fiber: 4g; Sugar: 3g; Protein: 21g; Iron: 1mg; Sodium: 402mg

Fluffy Blueberry Pancakes

Prep time: 5 minutes / *Cook time:* 10 minutes

Pancakes and waffles define Sunday mornings in many homes, and they can absolutely be a part of life with celiac disease. This recipe yields a light and fluffy cake. Pair with eggs or yogurt, as well as fruit such as fresh berries, for a satisfying meal.

1 large egg

2 tablespoons granulated sugar

2 tablespoons melted butter or vegetable oil, divided

1 teaspoon vanilla extract

1 cup all-purpose, gluten-free flour (Pillsbury works best for this recipe)

¼ teaspoon xanthan gum (if not already in flour)

1 tablespoon baking powder

¼ teaspoon salt

¾ cup milk

½ cup blueberries or 1 chopped banana (optional)

SERVES 8

30-MINUTE
NUT-FREE
VEGETARIAN

Ingredient Tip: To add more fiber, add in 1 tablespoon ground flax or chia seeds.

1. In a large bowl, whisk together the egg, sugar, 1 tablespoon of butter, and vanilla.

2. Mix in the gluten-free flour, xanthan gum (if using), baking powder, and salt. Stir in the milk until smooth.

3. In a griddle or sauté pan, melt the remaining 1 tablespoon of butter over medium heat.

4. Scoop ¼ cup batter onto the greased griddle or pan and cook in batches. Cook until the batter starts to bubble and puff. Flip and cook until golden brown.

5. Top with blueberries (if using) and enjoy!

Per Serving: Calories: 100; Total Fat: 3g; Saturated Fat: 1g; Carbohydrates: 15g; Fiber: 2g; Sugar: 4g; Protein: 3g; Iron: 0mg; Sodium: 100mg

Belgian-Style Waffles

Prep time: 15 minutes / *Cook time:* 10 minutes

Whether you're a waffle innovator, adding chicken and mashed potatoes, or prefer the more traditional track of butter and syrup, the crisp nooks and crannies of this recipe will set you up for a delicious meal. Enjoy these waffles with a protein, such as eggs or Greek yogurt, as well as a berry compote for the ultimate meal. You can also make a big batch of these waffles, freeze them, and then toast them when you need a quick breakfast.

1½ cups gluten-free flour

2 teaspoons baking powder

½ teaspoon salt

¾ cup whole milk

2 large eggs

5 tablespoons butter, melted

2 tablespoons maple syrup

1 teaspoon vanilla extract

Nonstick cooking spray

MAKES 6 LARGE WAFFLES

30-MINUTE

NUT-FREE

VEGETARIAN

1. In a mixing bowl, combine the flour, baking powder, and salt. In a separate bowl, whisk the milk, eggs, butter, maple syrup, and vanilla. Pour the wet ingredients into the dry and mix well. Let sit for 5 to 10 minutes.

2. Preheat a waffle iron to medium heat and spray with cooking spray.

3. Pour about ⅓ cup batter (or enough to cover the surface) onto the waffle iron and close the lid. Cook until golden brown, 3 to 5 minutes. Repeat with the remaining batter.

Substitution Tip: To make this dish dairy free, use a plant-based milk instead of cow's milk. While butter has no lactose, you can substitute that for melted coconut oil or vegetable oil.

Per Serving: Calories: 230; Total Fat: 13g; Saturated Fat: 7g; Carbohydrates: 22g; Fiber: 2g; Sugar: 6g; Protein: 6g; Iron: 1mg; Sodium: 297mg

Oatmeal Cakes with Cinnamon and Fruit

Prep time: 15 minutes / *Cook time:* 30 minutes

These oatmeal cakes combine the convenience of a muffin with the nutrition of oatmeal. It's a great chewy breakfast on the go or a nice midday snack. For a softer muffin, let the oats and milk soak for 2 hours, or as long as overnight, before combining the remaining ingredients and baking.

Nonstick cooking spray

2½ cups gluten-free rolled oats

1½ cups whole milk

1 large egg

⅓ cup maple syrup

2 tablespoons vegetable oil

1 teaspoon vanilla extract

1 teaspoon ground cinnamon

1 teaspoon baking powder

¼ teaspoon salt

⅓ cup dry cranberries (optional)

¾ cup fresh blueberries

MAKES 6 CAKES

NUT-FREE

VEGETARIAN

Ingredient Tip: For more fiber and heart-healthy fat, consider adding 2 tablespoons ground flaxseed or chia seeds or ½ cup of your favorite nuts or seeds, like pumpkin seeds or walnuts.

Substitution Tip: To make this dish oat-free, substitute 3 cups cooked quinoa for the oats and use 3 eggs instead of 1. Adding ¼ cup coconut flour will help hold the cakes together.

1. Preheat the oven to 375°F. Coat 6 cups of a muffin tin with cooking spray or use paper liners.

2. In a large bowl, mix the oats, milk, egg, maple syrup, oil, vanilla, cinnamon, baking powder, and salt until well combined. Fold in the cranberries (if using). Divide among the muffin cups, using ⅓ to ½ cup batter each. Top each cup with fresh blueberries.

3. Bake until firm, 25 to 30 minutes. Let cool for 10 minutes before removing from the tin. Serve warm.

Per Serving: Calories: 181; Total Fat: 7g; Saturated Fat: 2g; Carbohydrates: 25g; Fiber: 1g; Sugar: 15g; Protein: 5g; Iron: 1mg; Sodium: 41mg

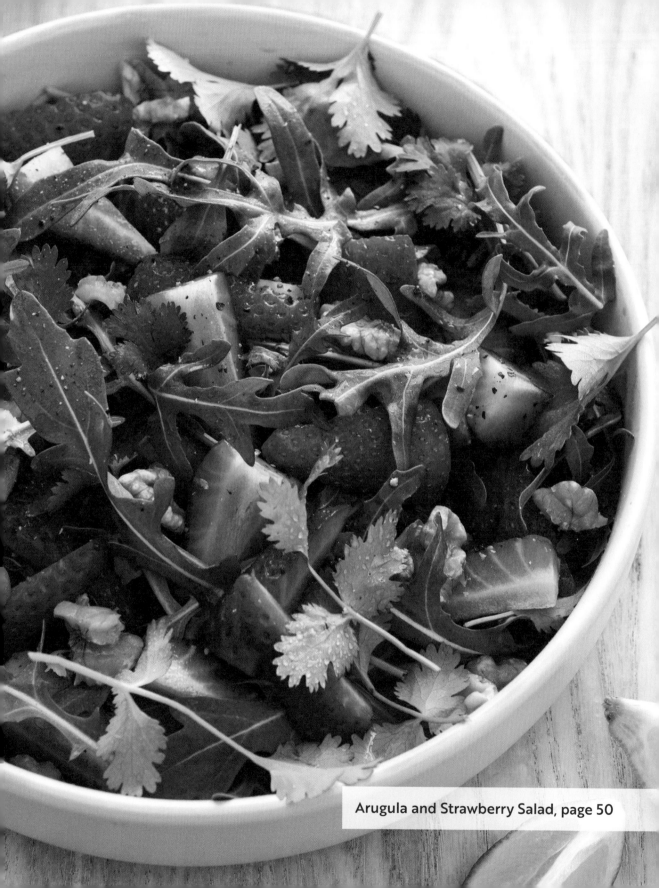

Arugula and Strawberry Salad, page 50

Salads and Soups

Arugula and Strawberry Salad

Prep time: 20 minutes

This refreshing summer salad goes great with grilled chicken, salmon, or beef. Serve with your favorite balsamic vinaigrette, balsamic glaze, or just lemon juice and olive oil.

4 cups arugula

1 cup sliced
fresh strawberries

½ cup sliced red onion

½ cup cashews, almonds,
or sesame seeds

⅓ cup dried cranberries

⅓ cup crumbled
feta cheese

Gluten-free balsamic
dressing or lime-based
dressing, for serving

SERVES 4

30-MINUTE

EGG-FREE

VEGETARIAN

Substitution Tip: Arugula has a peppery flavor and can have a short shelf life. For a mild flavor, try baby spinach or baby kale in place of or mixed with the arugula.

1. Place the arugula in a large bowl and layer the strawberries, onion, cashews, cranberries, and feta on top.

2. Dress with balsamic vinaigrette and serve.

Per Serving: Calories: 161; Total Fat: 10g; Saturated Fat: 4g; Carbohydrates: 12g; Fiber: 2g; Sugar: 4g; Protein: 6g; Iron: 2mg; Sodium: 167mg

Plump Tomato Caprese Salad

Prep time: 10 minutes

Caprese salad is a simple go-to that looks fancy! Serve alone as an appetizer or on top of your favorite gluten-free pasta for a delicious dish.

3 to 4 medium ripe tomatoes, cut into ¼-inch-thick slices or 2 cups halved cherry tomatoes

1 cucumber, peeled and cut into ¼-inch-thick rounds

1 pound fresh mozzarella cheese, cut into ¼-inch-thick rounds

½ cup packed fresh basil leaves

½ cup sliced red onion

Pinch garlic powder

Pinch sea salt

Pinch freshly ground black pepper

2 tablespoons extra-virgin olive oil

2 tablespoons balsamic glaze

SERVES 4

30-MINUTE
EGG-FREE
NUT-FREE
VEGETARIAN

Ingredient Tip: Tomatoes are a health-promoting powerhouse because of how much lycopene they contain, which is an antioxidant that has been linked to many health benefits, including reduced risk of heart disease and cancer. They also contain robust amounts of vitamin C, potassium, folate, and vitamin K.

1. On a serving platter, arrange the tomatoes, cucumber slices, and mozzarella.

2. Sprinkle the basil leaves, onion, garlic powder, salt, and pepper over the top.

3. Drizzle with the olive oil and balsamic glaze. Serve immediately.

Per Serving: Calories: 129; Total Fat: 8g; Saturated Fat: 2g; Carbohydrates: 11g; Fiber: 2g; Sugar: 6g; Protein: 4g; Iron: 1mg; Sodium: 51mg

Greek Spinach Salad

Prep time: 15 minutes

This salad is a shining example of how eating well is also delicious. The Mediterranean diet is consistently ranked as one of the healthiest ways to approach food, due to its heart-healthy fat content and wide rainbow of vegetables and fruits.

1 pint cherry or grape tomatoes, halved

1 red bell pepper, roughly chopped

1 yellow bell pepper, roughly chopped

1 cucumber, peeled, seeded, and cut into ¼-inch-thick slices

½ cup sliced red onion

½ cup pitted Kalamata olives

½ cup crumbled feta cheese

2 tablespoons red wine vinegar

Juice of ½ lemon

1 teaspoon dried oregano

Kosher salt

Freshly ground black pepper

¼ cup extra-virgin olive oil

4 cups baby spinach

SERVES 4

30-MINUTE
EGG-FREE
NUT-FREE
VEGETARIAN

Ingredient Tip: This Greek salad is packed with the heart-health benefits of olives and a vibrant rainbow of colors. Serve with grilled chicken, shrimp, or beef and a side of gluten-free pasta for a balanced meal.

1. In a large bowl, stir together the tomatoes, bell peppers, cucumber, red onion, and olives. Gently fold in the feta.

2. In a small bowl, combine the vinegar, lemon juice, and oregano and season with salt and pepper. Slowly whisk in the olive oil.

3. Place the spinach in a salad bowl and pour the other vegetables over the top.

4. Drizzle the dressing over the salad.

Per Serving: Calories: 226; Total Fat: 20g; Saturated Fat: 2g; Carbohydrates: 11g; Fiber: 2g; Sugar: 4g; Protein: 2g; Iron: 2mg; Sodium: 773mg

Avocado-Tuna Salad

Prep time: 5 minutes

Using avocado in place of mayonnaise is a fantastic way to make tuna salad the ultimate heart-healthy dish. If you enjoy toasted sandwiches, assemble it open-faced and bake or toast it for 5 minutes. For a heartier meal, serve topped with cheese, chopped tomatoes, bell pepper strips, and spinach.

1 avocado, pitted and peeled

1 (5-ounce) can water-packed tuna, drained

1 tablespoon chopped onion

1 teaspoon freshly squeezed lemon juice

Pinch garlic powder

Salt

Freshly ground black pepper

2 gluten-free wraps or 4 slices gluten-free bread

SERVES 2

30-MINUTE
DAIRY-FREE
EGG-FREE
NUT-FREE

Substitution Tip: Use canned or fresh chicken or cooked salmon instead of tuna for a change of flavor. If you don't have gluten-free bread or tortillas, use it as a dip along with your favorite gluten-free chips and raw vegetables.

1. In small bowl, mash the avocado.

2. Mix in the tuna, onion, lemon juice, and garlic powder. Season with salt and pepper.

3. Place half of the mixture on each wrap and serve.

Per Serving: Calories: 473; Total Fat: 30g; Saturated Fat: 6g; Carbohydrates: 30g; Fiber: 8g; Sugar: 3g; Protein: 27g; Iron: 2mg; Sodium: 410mg

Chili-Ginger Salmon over Spinach Salad

Prep time: 20 minutes, plus 20 minutes to marinate / *Cook time:* 10 minutes

This grilled salmon fillet over spinach salad is the perfect bite from beginning to end. The sweet fruit pairs perfectly with the savory salmon. Add a side of rice or quinoa to round out the dish. While this salmon tastes divine off the grill, if you don't have one, you can cook the salmon for 10 to 15 minutes under a hot broiler instead. Try this versatile salad with grilled tofu or tempeh for a vegetarian option, or with beef or chicken for a different flavor profile.

1 pound salmon fillet

4 tablespoons tamari

2 tablespoons brown sugar

2 tablespoons minced garlic or 1 teaspoon garlic powder

2 tablespoons minced and peeled fresh ginger or 1 teaspoon ground ginger

2 teaspoons sesame oil

2 teaspoons chili paste

4 cups baby spinach

½ cup shredded carrot

½ cup sliced cucumber

½ cup fresh blueberries

⅓ cup sliced red onion

⅓ cup crumbled feta cheese

⅓ cup chopped cashews

SERVES 4

EGG-FREE

Substitution Tip: To make this dish dairy free, simply leave out the feta cheese or use your favorite vegan feta cheese.

Substitution Tip: To save time, you can use a premade gluten-free sesame-ginger salad dressing to marinate the salmon, such as Annie's Organic Gluten-Free Sesame-Ginger Vinaigrette.

1. Place the salmon in a small baking dish.

2. In a small bowl, whisk the tamari, brown sugar, garlic, ginger, sesame oil, and chili paste. Set aside half of the mixture for dressing the salad later. Pour the remaining half over the salmon and marinate for 20 minutes.

3. In a large bowl, layer the spinach, carrot, cucumber, blueberries, onion, feta, and cashews.

4. Preheat a grill to medium-high heat and oil the grates of the grill.

5. Place the salmon on the grill. If there is skin, place the skinless side down first. Cover and grill for 4 to 6 minutes. Flip and grill for an additional 3 or 4 minutes. The salmon is done when it flakes easily with a fork. A 1-inch-thick fillet typically needs 6 to 10 minutes to cook.

6. Let the salmon rest for 5 minutes before serving on top of or alongside the salad.

Per Serving: Calories: 368; Total Fat: 22g; Saturated Fat: 5g; Carbohydrates: 16g; Fiber: 2g; Sugar: 9g; Protein: 28g; Iron: 3mg; Sodium: 750mg

Wild Rice Salad

Prep time: 15 minutes / *Cook time:* 15 minutes

This classic whole-grain salad has the perfect, satisfying texture paired with sweet and savory flavors that will leave you coming back for more. Pure wild rice takes a long time to cook. However, wild rice blends by Lundberg or RiceSelect provide similar flavor and texture with less time commitment.

3 cups cooked wild rice, cooled

1 cup halved green grapes

1 cup mandarin oranges segments

½ cup chopped scallions, both white and green parts, or chopped red onion

½ cup chopped pecans (optional)

¼ cup dried cranberries

½ cup orange juice (can use the juice from the mandarin oranges, if canned)

1 tablespoon extra-virgin olive oil

1 teaspoon garlic powder

½ teaspoon salt

¼ teaspoon freshly ground black pepper

SERVES 6

30-MINUTE
DAIRY-FREE
EGG-FREE
VEGAN

Substitution Tip: To bump up the protein and fiber content of this dish, consider adding 1½ cups of edamame beans or garbanzos.

1. In a large salad bowl, place the cooled wild rice, grapes, oranges, scallions, pecans (if using), and cranberries.

2. In a small bowl, mix the orange juice, olive oil, garlic powder, salt, and pepper. Pour the dressing over the wild rice salad. Toss together.

3. For more flavor, allow the salad to marinate in the refrigerator 30 to 45 minutes.

Per Serving: Calories: 211; Total Fat: 10g; Saturated Fat: 1g; Carbohydrates: 28g; Fiber: 3g; Sugar: 9g; Protein: 5g; Iron: 1mg; Sodium: 5mg

Chilled Quinoa Salad

Prep time: 15 minutes / *Cook time:* 20 minutes

This chilled quinoa salad is a refreshing crowd-pleaser for cookouts and summer grilling. Friends will be eager to get the recipe! Cook the rice in chicken broth instead of plain water for an extra level of rich flavor.

4 cups water or gluten-free chicken broth

2 cups quinoa, rinsed

¾ cup peeled chopped carrots

¾ cup halved cherry tomatoes

½ cup chopped cilantro

½ cup dry roasted sunflower seeds

¼ cup tamari

¼ cup freshly squeezed lemon juice

2 tablespoons extra-virgin olive oil

2 tablespoons minced garlic

Salt

Freshly ground black pepper

SERVES 6

DAIRY-FREE
EGG-FREE
NUT-FREE

Ingredient Tip: Quinoa is an ancient grain with a mild flavor. It cooks as fast and easily as rice but boasts over double the protein and fiber of rice.

1. In a medium pot, combine the water and quinoa. Bring to a boil over medium-high heat, then reduce the heat to a simmer for 15 minutes, until the grains have "popped" open and all the liquid is absorbed. Fluff with a fork and set aside to cool.

2. Once cool, pour into a large bowl and combine with the carrots, tomatoes, cilantro, sunflower seeds, tamari, lemon juice, olive oil, and garlic. Season with salt and pepper and mix well. Best served cold.

Per Serving: Calories: 288; Total Fat: 10g; Saturated Fat: 1g; Carbohydrates: 41g; Fiber: 5g; Sugar: 2g; Protein: 11g; Iron: 3mg; Sodium: 689mg

Thai Peanut-Quinoa Salad

Prep time: 15 minutes

This dish is the very definition of nourishing. High in protein, fiber, and iron, it can be eaten alone, but the color, flavor, and nutrients go so well with grilled salmon or chicken.

2 cups water

1 cup quinoa, rinsed

1 (15-ounce) can chickpeas, rinsed and drained

1 cup shredded purple cabbage

1 red bell pepper, chopped

½ cup shredded carrots

½ cup finely chopped cilantro

¼ cup finely chopped red onion

2 tablespoons peanut butter

2 tablespoons tamari

1 tablespoon minced garlic or ½ teaspoon garlic powder

1½ teaspoons grated and peeled fresh ginger or ½ teaspoon ground ginger

1 teaspoon apple cider vinegar or rice vinegar

¼ teaspoon ground cayenne pepper

Salt

Freshly ground black pepper

2 or 3 tablespoons warm water, to thin dressing

¼ cup crushed cashews, for garnish

SERVES 4

30-MINUTE
DAIRY-FREE
EGG-FREE
VEGAN

Allergen Tip: Use sunflower butter instead of peanut butter for the dressing, or if you prefer, try the salad without any nut butter. The combination of herbs and spices make this a flexible dish. To save time, use ½ cup of your favorite gluten-free peanut butter dressing.

1. In a medium pot, combine the water and quinoa. Bring to a boil over medium-high heat, then reduce the heat to a simmer for 15 minutes, until the liquid is absorbed and the grains have "popped" open. Fluff with a fork and allow to cool.

2. In a large bowl, combine the quinoa, chickpeas, cabbage, bell pepper, carrots, cilantro, and red onion.

3. In a small bowl, mix together the peanut butter, tamari, garlic, ginger, vinegar, and cayenne pepper. Season with salt and pepper. Mix to combine. Add water a tablespoon at a time, if necessary, to thin the mixture to a more dressing-like consistency. Pour over the salad and mix well to combine. Garnish with cashews.

Per Serving: Calories: 421; Total Fat: 9g; Saturated Fat: 1g; Carbohydrates: 66g; Fiber: 17g; Sugar: 13g; Protein: 21g; Iron: 11mg; Sodium: 589mg

Rice Noodle-Cabbage Salad

Prep time: 15 minutes / *Cook time:* 10 minutes

Ramen noodle-cabbage salad is a staple potluck dish at many midwestern events. This recipe is a great gluten-free spin on the old classic. You can use cashews or sesame seeds as garnish instead of the peanuts, if you like.

¼ cup tamari

¼ cup rice vinegar

2 tablespoons extra-virgin olive oil

2 tablespoons sesame oil

1 tablespoon minced garlic

2 teaspoons minced and peeled fresh ginger

7 ounces rice noodles

4 cups shredded purple cabbage

1 cup shredded carrots

½ cup chopped red onion

¼ cup chopped fresh cilantro

½ cup crushed peanuts

SERVES 6

30-MINUTE
DAIRY-FREE
EGG-FREE
VEGAN

Ingredient Tip: Purple fruits and vegetables such as cabbage are rich in anthocyanins. Studies have shown that anthocyanins may benefit brain health, reduce inflammation, and reduce the risk of cancer and heart disease.

1. In a large bowl, mix the tamari, vinegar, olive oil, sesame oil, garlic, and ginger.

2. Bring a large pot of water to a boil. Add the rice noodles and cook for 2 to 3 minutes, until al dente. Drain and rinse. Transfer the noodles to the bowl with the dressing. Toss to combine.

3. Add the cabbage, carrots, onions, and cilantro. Mix well.

4. Garnish with the crushed nuts. Enjoy immediately at room temperature or eat it cold after refrigerating. Store in an airtight container for up to 4 days in the refrigerator.

Per Serving: Calories: 224; Total Fat: 15g; Saturated Fat: 2g; Carbohydrates: 16g; Fiber: 3g; Sugar: 3g; Protein: 6g; Iron: 1mg; Sodium: 701mg

Chicken Vegetable Soup

Prep time: 15 minutes / *Cook time:* 45 minutes

Soup is perhaps one of the easiest recipes to prepare. Simply pair a protein with your favorite vegetables and broth for a dish that's sure to please.

2 tablespoons
  extra-virgin olive oil

2 cups chopped
  sweet potatoes
  (about 2 large
  sweet potatoes)

3 carrots, peeled
  and chopped

2 celery stalks, chopped

½ red onion, chopped

2 tablespoons
  minced garlic

1 pound chicken
  breasts, cut into
  bite-size cubes

6 cups water or
  chicken broth

1 teaspoon salt

2 bay leaves

Freshly ground
  black pepper

1 cup frozen peas

SERVES 8

DAIRY-FREE
EGG-FREE
NUT-FREE

Substitution Tip: This recipe calls for chicken but you can also use beef, ham, or even chickpeas, depending on your preference.

1. In a large pot, heat the olive oil over medium heat. Sauté the sweet potatoes, carrots, celery, onion, and garlic until fragrant, about 5 minutes. Add the chicken and sauté for 4 to 5 minutes, stirring regularly, until the chicken is browned.

2. Add the water, salt, bay leaves, and pepper and simmer for 25 to 30 minutes. Add the peas and cook another 10 minutes.

3. Remove the bay leaves before serving.

Per Serving: Calories: 187; Total Fat: 5g; Saturated Fat: 1g; Carbohydrates: 16g; Fiber: 3g; Sugar: 3g; Protein: 18g; Iron: 1mg; Sodium: 350mg

Soothing Chickpea, Carrot, and Coriander Soup

Prep time: 15 minutes / *Cook time:* 30 minutes

This carrot soup packs warmth into a cold day. Chickpeas blended into the mix add protein and fiber, as well as a thick, hearty texture. For a beautiful pop of color and flavor, you can also garnish the dish with cilantro.

4 tablespoons extra-virgin olive oil, divided

4 cups 2-inch pieces peeled and cut carrots

1 large red onion, chopped

2 tablespoons minced garlic

1 teaspoon ground coriander

Salt

Freshly ground black pepper

3 cups gluten-free reduced-sodium vegetable broth

3 cups water

1 (15-ounce) can chickpeas, drained and rinsed or 1½ cup cooked black beans

¼ cup packed minced fresh cilantro leaves, plus more for garnish

Pinch red pepper flakes

Lime wedges, for serving

SERVES 6

DAIRY-FREE
EGG-FREE
NUT-FREE
VEGAN

Ingredient Tip: Beans are an excellent source of fiber and protein, but many people fear them for their gas-producing properties. Rinsing beans before adding them to a dish can reduce this side effect. Most bodies can adjust to eating beans if eaten regularly. Start with small, consistent doses and work your way up.

Per Serving: Calories: 197;
Total Fat: 10g;
Saturated Fat: 2g;
Carbohydrates: 23g;
Fiber: 5g; Sugar: 5g;
Protein: 5g; Iron: 1mg;
Sodium: 895mg

1. In a large pot, heat 2 tablespoons of oil over medium-high heat and sauté the carrots, onion, garlic, and coriander. Season with salt and pepper. Cook until tender, about 8 minutes.

2. Add the broth, water, chickpeas, cilantro, and red pepper flakes. Bring to a boil, then reduce heat and let simmer for 15 minutes.

3. Using a blender or an immersion blender, blend until smooth. If using a blender, work in batches, being very careful when transferring the hot liquid.

4. Transfer to a bowl and serve with lime wedges.

Homestyle Slow Cooker Beef Stew

Prep time: 15 minutes / *Cook time:* 6 to 8 hours

Beef stew takes little time to prep but stew meat is tougher and needs time to tenderize over low heat. Prep it in the morning and cook in a slow cooker while you're away. You'll arrive home to a delicious, hearty meal.

¼ cup all-purpose gluten-free flour

1 pound beef stew meat, trimmed and cut into 1-inch cubes

2 tablespoons vegetable oil

5 medium carrots, peeled and cut into bite-size pieces

2 large baking potatoes, peeled and cut into ¾-inch cubes

3 cups beef broth

1 cup red wine

1 medium onion, chopped

1 (6-ounce) can tomato paste

2 tablespoons red wine vinegar

1 tablespoon gluten-free Worcestershire sauce

2 bay leaves

1 cup frozen peas

⅓ cup minced parsley

SERVES 8

DAIRY-FREE
EGG-FREE
NUT-FREE

Substitution Tip: If wine is unavailable, root beer is another excellent option to add flavor.

Per Serving: Calories: 281; Total Fat: 8g; Saturated Fat: 3g; Carbohydrates: 28g; Fiber: 5g; Sugar: 6g; Protein: 18g; Iron: 2mg; Sodium: 970mg

1. In a large bowl, toss the flour and beef to evenly coat. Heat the oil in a large skillet over medium-high heat. Brown the beef in small batches, about 5 minutes, until golden brown on each side.

2. Place the meat in the slow cooker along with the carrots, potatoes, broth, wine, onion, tomato paste, vinegar, Worcestershire sauce, and bay leaves. Cover and cook on low for 6 to 8 hours, or until the meat is tender. Stir in the frozen peas and half of the minced parsley. Use the remaining parsley as a garnish.

Butternut Squash Chili

Prep time: 20 minutes / *Cook time:* 1 hour

Cold winter days call for hearty soups. Butternut squash sweetens the pot while adding fiber and a variety of B vitamins.

2 tablespoons extra-virgin olive oil

1 medium red onion, chopped

1 red bell pepper, chopped

1 green bell pepper, chopped

1 small butternut squash, peeled and cut into ½-inch cubes

2 tablespoons minced garlic

1 tablespoon chili powder

1 teaspoon paprika

1 teaspoon ground cumin

½ teaspoon ground cayenne pepper

1 (15-ounce) can black beans, rinsed and drained or 1½ cups cooked black beans

1 (14.5-ounce) can diced tomatoes

1 (14.5-ounce) can tomato purée

1 cup vegetable broth

Salt

Freshly ground black pepper

¾ cup shredded sharp cheddar cheese or sour cream, for serving (optional)

SERVES 6

EGG-FREE
NUT-FREE

Ingredient Tip: Beans are an excellent source of iron, which is best absorbed when eaten with a source of vitamin C, such as tomatoes.

1. In a large pot, warm the olive oil over medium heat. Sauté the onion, bell peppers, butternut squash, and garlic. Cook while stirring occasionally, until fragrant.

2. Reduce the heat down to medium-low and add the chili powder, paprika, cumin, and cayenne. Cook, stirring regularly, for about 30 seconds. Add the black beans, tomatoes and their juices, tomato purée, and broth. Stir to combine and cover for about 1 hour, stirring occasionally.

3. You'll know the chili is done when the butternut squash is tender and the liquid has reduced a bit. Garnish each bowl with about 2 tablespoons cheddar cheese or sour cream (if using) and serve.

Per Serving: Calories: 171; Total Fat: 5g; Saturated Fat: 1g; Carbohydrates: 26g; Fiber: 7g; Sugar: 8g; Protein: 7g; Iron: 2mg; Sodium: 240mg

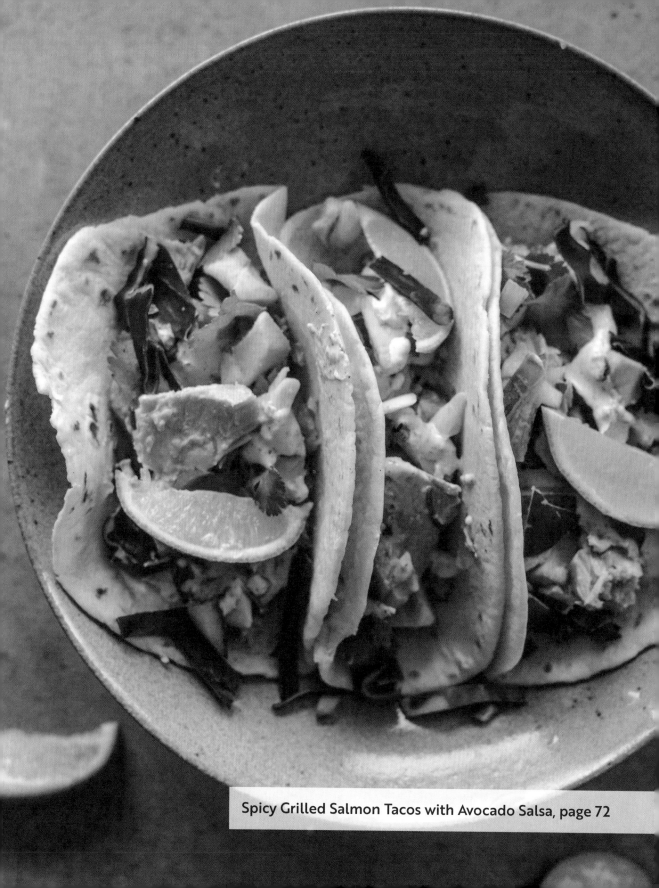

Spicy Grilled Salmon Tacos with Avocado Salsa, page 72

Seafood and Meat

Shrimp Scampi with Zoodles

Prep time: 5 minutes / *Cook time:* 12 minutes

Zucchini noodles are ready in a flash, adding a burst of fiber and nutrients to this traditional dish. If you don't have a spiralizer, use a cheese shredder for a shorter, yet equally delicious noodle.

6 tablespoons butter

⅓ red onion, chopped

4 garlic cloves, minced

½ teaspoon red pepper flakes

½ cup vegetable broth

1 tablespoon freshly squeezed lemon juice

1½ pounds medium shrimp, peeled and deveined

Salt

Freshly ground black pepper

6 cups zucchini noodles (about 2 zucchinis)

¼ cup roughly chopped, fresh flat-leaf parsley

SERVES 4

30-MINUTE
EGG-FREE
NUT-FREE

Prep Ahead Tip: Vegetable noodles can be spiralized or shredded 3 to 4 days in advance. Simply spiralize or shred your favorite vegetables (zucchini, beets, or butternut squash) and store in an airtight container until you're ready to cook them.

1. In a large sauté pan or skillet, melt the butter over medium-high heat. Add the onion, garlic, and red pepper flakes. Cook until fragrant and the garlic is just golden, about 2 minutes. Add the broth and lemon juice. Cook until golden, 4 to 5 minutes. Add the shrimp, salt, and pepper and cook, stirring frequently, until the shrimp turns pink, about 3 minutes.

2. Add the zucchini noodles and toss with tongs until they are slightly wilted and coated with sauce, about 3 minutes. Season with salt and pepper.

3. Transfer to a serving bowl and sprinkle with parsley.

Per Serving: Calories: 343; Total Fat: 19g; Saturated Fat: 11g; Carbohydrates: 5g; Fiber: 1g; Sugar: 2g; Protein: 38g; Iron: 6mg; Sodium: 614mg

Sweet and Spicy Shrimp Kebabs

Prep time: 10 minutes / *Cook time:* 10 minutes

These sweet and spicy kebabs are a fantastic reason to get out of the kitchen on a hot summer day. They're easy to prepare and ready in a flash. If you are using wood skewers, be sure to soak the skewers in water for 15 minutes before grilling. Pair with a bowl of rice for a delicious meal.

3 tablespoons sesame oil

3 tablespoons freshly squeezed lime juice

2 tablespoons chopped fresh cilantro

1 tablespoon honey

½ teaspoon salt

12 jumbo raw shrimp, peeled and deveined

3 jalapeño peppers, stemmed, seeded and quartered lengthwise

3 plums, pitted and cut into quarters

SERVES 4

30-MINUTE
DAIRY-FREE
EGG-FREE
NUT-FREE

1. Preheat the grill to medium-high.

2. In a large bowl, whisk the sesame oil, lime juice, cilantro, honey, and salt. Set aside 3 tablespoons of the mixture in a small bowl to use as a dressing. To the remaining marinade, add the shrimp, jalapeños, and plums and toss to coat.

3. Onto 4 (10-inch) skewers, thread the shrimp, jalapeños, and plums, evenly alternating between the skewers.

4. Grill the kebabs for 8 minutes, turning once halfway through. Drizzle with the reserved dressing.

Per Serving: Calories: 208; Total Fat: 11g; Saturated Fat: 2g; Carbohydrates: 11g; Fiber: 1g; Sugar: 11g; Protein: 15g; Iron: 1mg; Sodium: 452mg

Substitution Tip: If you are not fond of shrimp, this recipe can also be made with chicken. If using chicken, grill for 10 to 14 minutes total, turning once halfway through. If you do not have a grill, turn the oven to broil and move the top rack 5 inches from the top. Once the kebabs are assembled, broil on the top rack, 2 to 3 minutes each side. If using chicken, broil 4 to 8 minutes each side.

Savory Tuna Patties

Prep time: 10 minutes / *Cook time:* 10 minutes

Canned tuna is a convenient source of protein. Tuna patties are a great way to change up your tuna sandwich routine with a hot dish. Serve on Gluten-Free Bread (page 118) with lettuce, tomato, and onion or on top of your favorite garden salad.

2 (5-ounce) cans water-packed tuna, drained

½ cup almond flour

1 tablespoon minced garlic or 1 teaspoon garlic powder

1 teaspoon paprika

1 tablespoon freshly squeezed lemon juice

2 tablespoons grated red onion

1½ teaspoons Dijon mustard or mustard powder

1 large egg

½ teaspoon freshly ground black pepper

¼ teaspoon salt

1 tablespoon extra-virgin olive oil

SERVES 6

30-MINUTE

DAIRY-FREE

Substitution Tip: If tuna isn't your favorite fish, you can use the same recipe with canned salmon or chicken.

1. In a medium bowl, combine the tuna, almond flour, garlic, paprika, lemon juice, red onion, mustard, egg, pepper, and salt. Stir until mixed well. If the mixture won't stick together, allow it to sit in the refrigerator for 20 minutes.

2. When ready to cook, in a cast iron skillet, heat the olive oil over medium heat. Once the pan is hot, form the tuna mixture into 6 patties and cook in the oil for 4 minutes each side, until golden.

Per Serving: Calories: 156; Total Fat: 9g; Saturated Fat: 2g; Carbohydrates: 1g; Fiber: 0g; Sugar: 0g; Protein: 177g; Iron: 1mg; Sodium: 138mg

Grilled Spicy Salmon with Rub

Prep time: 5 minutes / *Cook time:* 12 minutes

With this recipe, salmon goes from refrigerator to table in less than 15 minutes for an easy and convenient dose of heart-healthy fat. Pair this dish with brown rice or quinoa and steamed broccoli for the perfect balance of nutrients. If you don't have a grill, broil the salmon for 10 to 12 minutes instead.

2 tablespoons packed
    light brown sugar

1 tablespoon
    minced garlic

1 tablespoon
    chili powder

1 teaspoon ground cumin

⅛ teaspoon salt

⅛ teaspoon freshly
    ground black pepper

2 pounds skinless,
    boneless salmon

1 tablespoon extra-virgin
    olive oil

SERVES 4

30-MINUTE
DAIRY-FREE
EGG-FREE
NUT-FREE

1. Coat your grill or a grill pan with oil and preheat over medium heat. While the grill is heating, in a small bowl, combine the brown sugar, garlic, chili powder, cumin, salt, and pepper. Brush the salmon with olive oil and rub with the spice mixture.

2. Grill the salmon for 4 to 5 minutes. Flip and cook for another 5 to 6 minutes for medium. For more well-done fish, cook an additional 1 to 2 minutes. Remove from the grill and serve immediately to avoid continued cooking.

Prep Ahead Tip: Preparing your own spice mixes is a great way to simplify meal prep. Simply combine your preferred spices and store in an airtight container in a cool, dry space. Empty spice bottles are the perfect fit! This spice mix goes well with salmon, chicken, and roasted vegetables.

Per Serving: Calories: 365; Total Fat: 17g; Saturated Fat: 3g; Carbohydrates: 9g; Fiber: 0g; Sugar: 9g; Protein: 44g; Iron: 2mg; Sodium: 176mg

Spicy Grilled Salmon Tacos with Avocado Salsa

Prep time: 20 minutes / *Cook time:* 6 minutes

Salmon is seasoned brilliantly with Mexican spices, then grilled for a crisp finish. It all comes together in a perfect package, topped with refreshing avocado salsa and crunchy tortilla chips.

For the Salmon

1 tablespoon extra-virgin olive oil, plus more for grill

1 tablespoon freshly squeezed lime juice

1 tablespoon minced garlic

1 teaspoon ancho chili powder

¾ teaspoon ground cumin

½ teaspoon paprika

½ teaspoon ground coriander

1½ pounds salmon

For the Avocado Salsa

2 medium avocados, peeled, cored, and chopped

½ cup frozen corn, thawed

½ cup cooked black beans

⅓ cup chopped red onion

3 tablespoons chopped cilantro

1 tablespoon minced garlic

2 tablespoons freshly squeezed lime juice

Salt

Freshly ground black pepper

For the Tacos

4 gluten-free corn tortillas or cooked rice, for serving

1 to 2 cups shredded purple cabbage, for serving

1 cup shredded sharp cheddar cheese, for serving (optional)

SERVES 4

**30-MINUTE
EGG-FREE
NUT-FREE**

Substitution Tip: Tacos don't have to be in a tortilla. This recipe also goes well served over a bed of rice or quinoa with a crumble of chips for texture.

1. Preheat a gas grill over medium-high heat and oil the grill surface.

2. In a mixing bowl, whisk together the olive oil, lime juice, garlic, ancho chili powder, cumin, onion powder, paprika, and coriander. Rub the mixture over the salmon. Place the salmon on the grill and cook, rotating once halfway through cooking, until cooked through, about 3 minutes per side.

3. Meanwhile, in a mixing bowl, gently toss together the avocado, corn, black beans, red onion, cilantro, garlic, and lime juice. Season with salt and pepper.

4. Break the salmon into small portions and layer over the center of the tortillas. Add the cabbage, avocado salsa, and sharp cheddar cheese, if using. Serve warm.

Per Serving: Calories: 379; Total Fat: 18g; Saturated Fat: 3g; Carbohydrates: 25g; Fiber: 8g; Sugar: 4g; Protein: 30g; Iron: 3mg; Sodium: 54mg

Jambalaya

Prep time: 15 minutes / *Cook time:* 40 minutes

Jambalaya is a versatile dish exploding with flavor. This one-pot meal will warm up a brisk fall day. Experiment with your favorite vegetables—such as peppers, mushrooms, zucchini, carrots, and squash—for the perfect bite.

3 tablespoons extra-virgin olive oil

2 boneless, skinless chicken breasts, cut into 1-inch cubes

1 pound chicken sausage, thinly sliced

3 bell peppers, chopped

1 white onion, chopped

1 jalapeño pepper, seeded and finely chopped

2 tablespoons minced garlic

1 pound raw medium shrimp, peeled and deveined

3 cups chicken stock

1 (14.5-ounce) can crushed tomatoes

1½ cups long-grain white rice

1 teaspoon crushed dried thyme

½ teaspoon dried oregano

½ teaspoon paprika

¼ teaspoon cayenne pepper

1 bay leaf

SERVES 8

DAIRY-FREE
EGG-FREE
NUT-FREE

Substitution Tip: Customize with any combination of your favorite proteins, such as chicken, shrimp, or sausage. If you prefer the dish without meat, add crumbled tempeh and/ or a few cups of black beans for protein.

Per Serving: Calories: 369; Total Fat: 12g; Saturated Fat: 3g; Carbohydrates: 37g; Fiber: 4g; Sugar: 6g; Protein: 29g; Iron: 4mg; Sodium: 789mg

1. In a large pot, heat the olive oil over medium-high heat. Add the chicken, chicken sausage, bell peppers, onion, jalapeño, and garlic. Sauté for 5 to 6 minutes, stirring occasionally, until the sausage is brown and the onions have softened.

2. Add the shrimp, chicken stock, tomatoes and their juices, rice, thyme, oregano, paprika, cayenne, and bay leaf and stir to combine. Reduce the heat to medium-low, cover, and simmer for 25 to 30 minutes, or until the rice is nearly cooked through, stirring every 5 minutes so that the rice does not burn. Remove and discard the bay leaf before serving.

Spiced Peach Chicken

Prep time: 10 minutes / *Cook time:* 25 minutes

The sweet and spicy combo is perfect in this recipe. Pair this simple baked chicken with rice or quinoa and steamed green beans for a colorful, nourishing meal.

1 cup canned diced peaches in syrup

1 jalapeño pepper, seeded and minced

1 tablespoon extra-virgin olive oil

1 tablespoon minced garlic

1 teaspoon ground paprika

Salt

Freshly ground black pepper

2 boneless, skinless chicken breasts

SERVES 2

DAIRY-FREE
EGG-FREE
NUT-FREE

Substitution Tip: If you prefer a less sweet dish, use canned peaches in juice and drain before adding to the recipe.

1. Preheat the oven to 400°F. Grease an 8-by-8-inch baking dish and set aside.

2. In a medium bowl, combine the peaches and syrup, jalapeño, olive oil, garlic, and paprika. Season with salt and pepper.

3. Place the chicken in the baking dish. Pour the fruit mixture over the top.

4. Bake for 25 to 30 minutes or until the internal temperature of the chicken reads 165°F and juices run clear.

Per Serving: Calories: 212; Total Fat: 8g; Saturated Fat: 1g; Carbohydrates: 7g; Fiber: 1g; Sugar: 7g; Protein: 26g; Iron: 1mg; Sodium: 75mg

Buffalo Chicken-Tater Tot Casserole

Prep time: 15 minutes / *Cook time:* 35 minutes

Buffalo sauce adds a zest to the classic tater tot casserole. It's great fuel to cheer on your favorite sports team!

2 tablespoons
   extra-virgin olive oil

½ cup chopped celery

⅓ onion, chopped

1 tablespoon
   minced garlic

1 (12-ounce) can
   gluten-free cream of
   celery soup (such as
   Pacific Foods)

2 cups cooked
   chopped chicken

1 cup shredded sharp
   cheddar cheese

1 bell pepper, chopped

½ cup sour cream or
   cream cheese

½ cup whole milk

½ cup buffalo sauce

½ cup crumbled
   blue cheese

1 (16-ounce) package
   tater tots

SERVES 12

EGG-FREE

NUT-FREE

Substitution Tip: If you don't like buffalo sauce, skip it and instead add ¼ cup milk for a hearty casserole.

Ingredient Tip: To make your own buffalo sauce, in a saucepan over medium heat, combine ½ cup hot sauce, ¼ cup cold unsalted butter, 1 tablespoon white vinegar, ¼ teaspoon ground cayenne pepper, and ⅛ teaspoon garlic powder. Bring to a simmer while stirring with a whisk. Once it starts to bubble on the sides of the pan, remove from the heat.

1. Preheat the oven to 400°F. Grease an 8-by-8-inch baking dish and set aside.

2. In a medium sauté pan or skillet, heat the olive oil over medium-high heat. Add the celery, onion, and garlic. Cook until fragrant.

3. In a large bowl, combine the soup, chicken, cheese, cooked vegetables, bell pepper, sour cream, milk, buffalo sauce, and blue cheese.

4. Pour the mixture into the prepared baking dish. Top with the tater tots.

5. Cover with foil and bake for 20 minutes. Remove the foil and bake uncovered for 15 minutes more to slightly crisp up the cheese on top.

6. Let stand for 5 minutes before serving.

Per Serving: Calories: 229; Total Fat: 14g; Saturated Fat: 6g; Carbohydrates: 15g; Fiber:2g;Sugar:2g;Protein:11g; Iron: 1mg; Sodium: 574mg

Honey Pork Tenderloin

Prep time: 15 minutes / *Cook time:* 50 minutes

This pork tenderloin is delicious enough for fancy occasions and healthy enough to eat every night. Serve with mashed potatoes or rice along with your favorite steamed or roasted vegetables for the perfect meal.

2 pounds
   pork tenderloin

¼ cup tamari

3 tablespoons honey

3 tablespoons
   extra-virgin olive oil

2 tablespoons
   orange juice

2 tablespoons
   Dijon mustard

2 tablespoons
   minced garlic

2 teaspoons
   dried rosemary

Salt

Freshly ground
   black pepper

SERVES 8

DAIRY-FREE
EGG-FREE
NUT-FREE

Ingredient Tip: Pork tenderloin is just as lean as white meat chicken. It offers a nice change of pace and flavor for those trying to eat well. For extra flavor, marinate the pork tenderloin for 1 hour prior to cooking. Simply place the meat in a large, resealable plastic bag with seasonings and store in the refrigerator until ready to cook.

1. Preheat the oven to 350°F. Line a baking sheet with parchment paper or grease with oil.

2. Place the pork tenderloin on the prepared baking sheet and cut 2-inch slits along the length of it.

3. In a small bowl, whisk together the tamari, honey, olive oil, orange juice, Dijon mustard, garlic, rosemary, salt, and pepper. Pour the sauce over the top of the pork.

4. Bake for 40 to 50 minutes, spooning the sauce over the top of the tenderloin every 10 minutes. Bake until a thermometer inserted in the center reads 145°F or the juices run clear.

5. Remove the tenderloin from the oven and allow to rest for 10 minutes before slicing and serving.

Per Serving: Calories: 238; Total Fat: 9g; Saturated Fat: 2g; Carbohydrates: 7g; Fiber: 0g; Sugar: 7g; Protein: 30g; Iron: 2mg; Sodium: 568mg

Southern-Style Pulled Pork

Prep time: 5 minutes / *Cook time:* 4 to 8 hours

Pulled pork is simple to prepare and an easy crowd-pleaser. It's the perfect dish when hosting gatherings for those with or without celiac disease.

3 pounds boneless pork
  roast, trimmed

1 (15-ounce) can
  tomato sauce

1 cup chicken or
  beef broth

1 (6-ounce) can
  tomato paste

⅔ cup brown sugar

½ cup apple
  cider vinegar

⅓ cup minced red onion

1 tablespoon
  garlic powder

1 teaspoon
  mustard powder

1 tablespoon freshly
  squeezed lemon juice

SERVES 16

DAIRY-FREE
EGG-FREE
NUT-FREE

Substitution Tip: Chicken breasts make a great substitute for those looking for another white meat.

1. Place the pork roast in a slow cooker.

2. In a medium bowl, combine the tomato sauce, broth, tomato paste, brown sugar, apple cider vinegar, onion, garlic powder, mustard powder, and lemon juice. Pour the mixture over the pork roast.

3. Cover and cook on low for 7 to 8 hours or on high for 4 hours, until the meat shreds easily.

4. Use two forks to shred the pork, either in the slow cooker or on a cutting board.

5. Serve as-is or on a gluten-free roll.

Per Serving: Calories: 153; Total Fat: 3g; Saturated Fat: 1g; Carbohydrates: 7g; Fiber: 0g; Sugar: 8g; Protein: 22g; Iron: 1mg; Sodium: 237mg

Mini Spicy Meatloaf Muffins

Prep time: 15 minutes / *Cook time:* 40 minutes

Meatloaf muffins are a great way to make meatloaf exciting. This dish adds a bit of zest using enchilada sauce instead of traditional tomato. Serve with rice, extra quinoa, or mashed potatoes, as well as a salad or veggie side for a balanced meal.

Nonstick cooking spray (optional)

1 teaspoon extra-virgin olive oil

1 red bell pepper, finely chopped

½ cup chopped onion

2 tablespoons minced garlic

⅔ cup cooked quinoa

½ cup tomato sauce

1 teaspoon ground cumin

1 teaspoon dried oregano

1 teaspoon chili powder

Salt

Freshly ground black pepper

1 pound lean ground turkey breast

⅔ cup shredded sharp cheddar cheese, divided

1 large egg

SERVES 6

NUT-FREE

Make Ahead Tip: These meatloaf muffins freeze well after baking for an easy addition to future meals. Simply allow to fully cool before storing in an airtight container. Freeze for up to 4 weeks and reheat in the oven or toaster oven.

Per Serving: Calories: 228; Total Fat: 12g; Saturated Fat: 5g; Carbohydrates: 10g; Fiber: 2g; Sugar: 2g; Protein: 19g; Iron: 4mg; Sodium: 164mg

1. Preheat the oven to 350°F. Spray a 12-cup muffin tin with cooking spray or line with muffin liners.

2. In a medium sauté pan or skillet, heat the olive oil over medium heat. Add the bell pepper, onion, and garlic and cook until fragrant, 3 to 5 minutes.

3. In a large bowl, combine the cooked vegetables with the quinoa, tomato sauce, cumin, oregano, and chili powder. Season with salt and pepper.

4. Stir in the ground turkey, ⅓ cup of cheese, and the egg. Mix well.

5. Add ¼ cup of the meatloaf mixture to each muffin cup. Sprinkle the remaining ⅓ cup of cheese over the top of the muffins.

6. Bake for 30 to 35 minutes. Let cool for a few minutes, then serve.

Ham and Cheese Casserole

Prep time: 20 minutes / *Cook time:* 35 minutes

Casseroles are a gift for busy people. Simply combine your favorite grains, protein, and vegetables with a cream soup and voila! It's dinner.

2 tablespoons extra-virgin olive oil

½ cup chopped celery

⅓ onion, chopped

1 tablespoon minced garlic

2 cups cooked gluten-free pasta (such as Banza)

1 (12-ounce) can gluten-free cream of celery soup (such as Pacific Foods)

1½ cups chopped ham

½ cup sour cream or cream cheese

½ cup whole milk

1½ cups shredded sharp cheddar cheese, divided

SERVES 8

EGG-FREE

NUT-FREE

Substitution Tip: Use your favorite protein source in this quick and easy casserole, such as ham, chicken, or tuna. If you prefer it without meat, add 2 cups of chickpeas for a delicious meat-free meal.

1. Preheat the oven to 400°F. Grease an 8-by-8-inch baking dish and set aside.

2. In a medium sauté pan or skillet, heat the olive oil over medium-high heat. Add the celery, onion, and garlic. Cook until fragrant.

3. In a large bowl, combine the pasta, soup, cooked vegetables, ham, sour cream, milk, and ¾ cup of cheese. Stir well to combine.

4. Pour the mixture into the prepared baking dish. Top with the remaining ¾ cup of cheese.

5. Cover with aluminum foil and bake for 20 minutes. Remove the foil and bake uncovered for 15 minutes to slightly crisp up the cheese on top.

6. Let stand for 5 minutes serving.

Per Serving: Calories: 300; Total Fat: 20g; Saturated Fat: 8g; Carbohydrates: 18g; Fiber: 4g; Sugar: 4g; Protein: 16g; Iron: 3mg; Sodium: 826mg

Ginger Beef and Broccoli

Prep time: 15 minutes / *Cook time:* 15 minutes

Beef and broccoli is a staple at most Asian-inspired restaurants. But the use of soy sauce often means it has gluten. Preparing it at home using tamari or Bragg Liquid Aminos is a simple way to make it gluten-free without sacrificing flavor. This dish pairs well with rice.

For the Beef

2 teaspoons tamari

¼ teaspoon sugar

¼ teaspoon salt

¾ pound boneless sirloin, cut across the grain into ¼-inch-thick slices

For the Sauce

1 tablespoon cornstarch

1 tablespoon tamari or Bragg Liquid Aminos

¼ cup chicken broth, beef broth, or water

2 teaspoons sesame oil

1 teaspoon sugar

3 tablespoons vegetable oil, divided

1 tablespoon minced and peeled fresh ginger or 1 teaspoon ground ginger

1 tablespoon minced garlic or 1 teaspoon garlic powder

1 pound fresh broccoli florets, chopped into bite-size pieces

⅓ cup water

SERVES 2

30-MINUTE
DAIRY-FREE
EGG-FREE
NUT-FREE

Ingredient Tip: When stir-frying beef, it's best to use a tender cut. Sirloin, tri-tip, rib eye, top loin (strip), tenderloin, shoulder center, and shoulder top blade are ideal.

1. To make the beef, in a small bowl, stir together the tamari, sugar, and salt. Add the beef and let it marinate for 20 minutes.

2. To make the sauce, while the beef is marinating, in a separate small bowl, dissolve the cornstarch in the tamari. Stir in the broth, sesame oil, and sugar.

continued ➤

3. In a wok or large skillet, heat 2 tablespoons of vegetable oil over high heat. In small batches, sauté the beef until no longer pink, about 1 minute. Transfer to a plate and set aside.

4. Add the remaining 1 tablespoon of vegetable oil to the wok and heat until hot. Stir-fry the ginger and garlic until fragrant, about 30 seconds. Add the broccoli and stir-fry for 1 minute. Add the water and steam the broccoli, covered, until it is crisp-tender, 2 to 3 minutes. Add the beef and sauce to the wok and stir-fry another 2 minutes, or until the sauce is thickened. Serve.

Per Serving: Calories: 295; Total Fat: 15g; Saturated Fat: 6g; Carbohydrates: 9g; Fiber: 2g; Sugar: 2g; Protein: 26g; Iron: 1mg; Sodium: 500mg

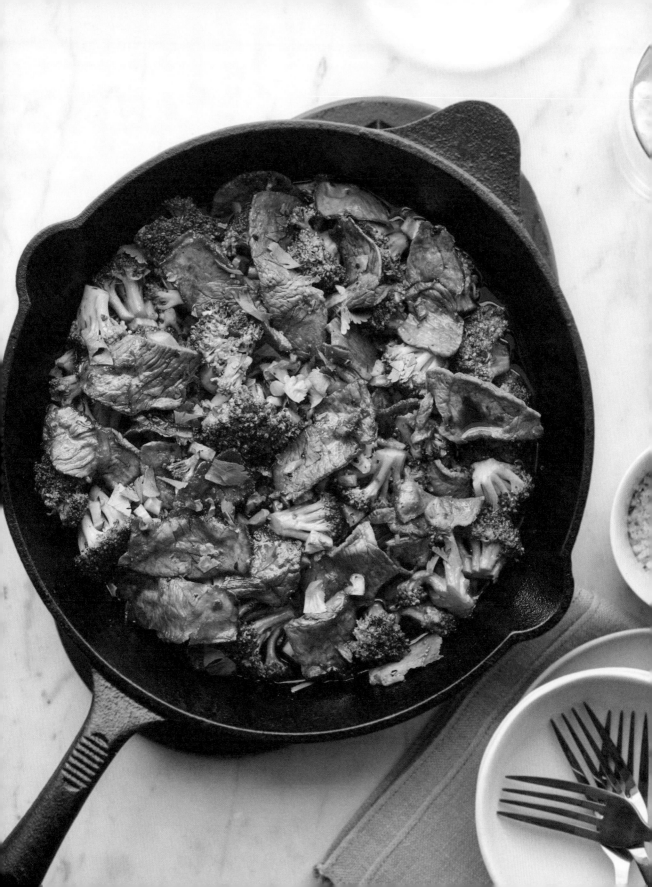

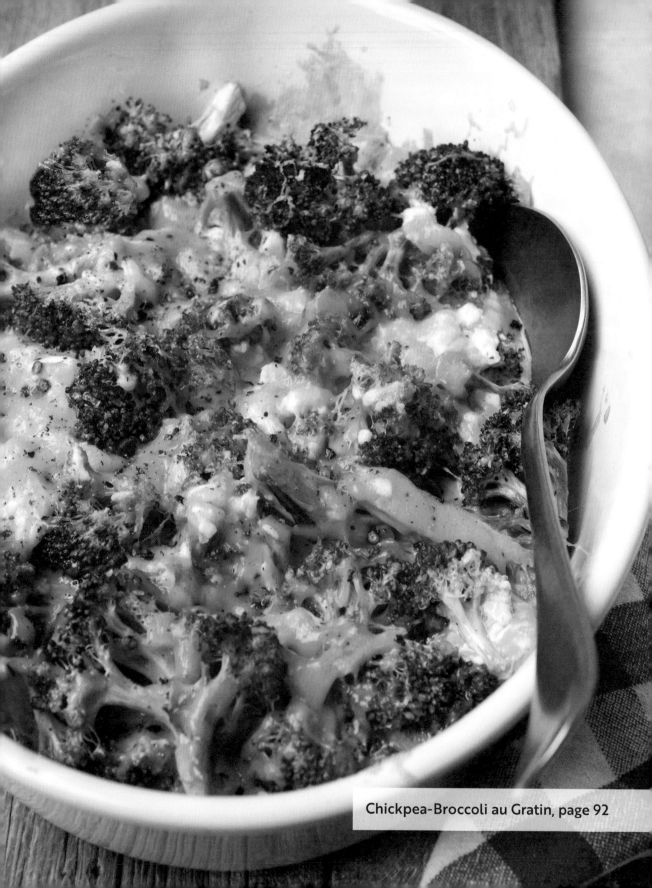

Chickpea-Broccoli au Gratin, page 92

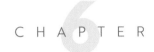

CHAPTER 6

Vegetarian and Vegan

Crispy Tofu Tacos with Pickled Vegetables

Prep time: 10 minutes / *Cook time:* 8 minutes

This tofu recipe showcases the Asian-Mexican fusion tacos that have grown popular in recent years. With bright colors and a crisp finish, quick pickled vegetables create a bite that's sure to please.

To Make the Pickled Vegetables

½ cup chopped red onion

½ cup shredded carrot

½ cup shredded cabbage

½ cup peeled, seeded, and chopped cucumber

½ cup rice vinegar

3 tablespoons freshly squeezed lime juice

2 tablespoons tamari

1 tablespoon sugar

Salt

Freshly ground black pepper

To Make the Greek Yogurt Dressing

⅓ cup Greek yogurt

1 tablespoon chili powder

To Make the Tofu

14 ounces tofu, drained and pressed

¼ cup cornstarch

1 teaspoon garlic powder

2 tablespoons vegetable oil

8 corn tortillas, for serving

½ cup chopped fresh cilantro, for serving

SERVES 4

30-MINUTE

EGG-FREE

NUT-FREE

VEGETARIAN

Make Ahead Tip: Pickled vegetables are designed to last and are more flavorful with time. Combine your favorite vegetables with rice vinegar in a mason jar. Store in the refrigerator and add to your favorite dishes for up to a week.

1. To make the pickled vegetables, in a medium bowl, combine the onion, carrot, cabbage, cucumber, rice vinegar, lime juice, tamari, and sugar. Season with salt and pepper. Let stand at least 15 minutes.

2. To make the Greek yogurt dressing, in a separate small bowl, whisk together the yogurt and chili powder and set aside.

3. Slice the tofu into ½-inch-thick slabs. In a gallon resealable plastic bag, combine the cornstarch and garlic powder and season with salt and pepper. Add the tofu and gently toss to coat.

4. In a large sauté pan or skillet, heat the oil over medium-high heat. Add the tofu and cook until crispy and light golden brown, about 4 minutes on each side. Transfer to a paper towel–lined plate.

5. Serve the tofu warm in corn tortillas with the pickled vegetables, Greek yogurt dressing, and fresh cilantro.

Per Serving: Calories: 300; Total Fat: 13g; Saturated Fat: 3g; Carbohydrates: 31g; Fiber: 5g; Sugar: 6g; Protein: 16g; Iron: 2mg; Sodium: 70mg

Caprese Pizza

Prep time: 30 minutes / *Cook time:* 20 to 30 minutes

This delicious pizza comes out crisp and delicious as a thin-crust pizza. Use a light variety of your favorite toppings or the caprese recipe below.

For the Crust

¾ cup warm water (about 100°F)

2 teaspoons sugar

1 teaspoon instant or active dry yeast

2 cups gluten-free baking flour, such as King Arthur Measure for Measure or Bob's Red Mill

¼ cup extra-virgin olive oil

1 teaspoon apple cider vinegar

1 teaspoon salt

For the Pizza

1 cup shredded mozzarella

10 cherry tomatoes, halved

⅓ red onion, sliced

Large handful fresh basil leaves

1 teaspoon garlic powder

SERVES 8

EGG-FREE
NUT-FREE
VEGETARIAN

To Make the Crust

1. In a small bowl, combine the warm water, sugar, and yeast. Let stand and allow to foam until it doubles in size, about 10 minutes.

2. In a separate bowl or using a food processor, mix together the flour, olive oil, vinegar, salt, and yeast mixture. Continuc to mix until the dough is smooth and elastic.

3. Cover the dough with a damp towel or plastic wrap and let rise in a warm place until the dough has puffed slightly, about 20 minutes. It will not rise as dramatically as conventional dough.

4. Preheat the oven to 400°F. Line a nonstick baking sheet with parchment paper or lightly grease with oil. With greased fingers, spread the dough to cover the pan.

5. Bake the dough for 10 minutes, then carefully remove it from the oven.

To Make the Pizza

Top the crust with the mozzarella, tomatoes, onions, basil leaves, and garlic. Bake another 10 to 15 minutes, until the cheese is melted. Enjoy hot!

Per Serving: Calories: 213; Total Fat: 10g; Saturated Fat: 3g; Carbohydrates: 23g; Fiber: 2g; Sugar: 2g; Protein: 7g; Iron: 1mg; Sodium: 101mg

Curried Waldorf Tofu Salad

Prep time: 5 minutes

This curry salad is an inspired twist on the traditional Waldorf salad's combination of apples and grapes. While this vegetarian version calls for tofu, it can also be made with shredded or canned chicken. Mango chutney is a sweet and savory condiment that can be found in most major grocery stores, typically by the salsa and other international foods.

½ cup plain Greek yogurt

2 tablespoons prepared mango chutney

2 teaspoons yellow curry powder

Salt

Freshly ground black pepper

7 ounces tofu, drained and pressed, then crumbled

½ cup chopped celery

½ cup halved red grapes

½ green apple, chopped

¼ cup chopped red onion

Romaine lettuce or gluten-free wraps, for serving

SERVES 2

30-MINUTE
EGG-FREE
NUT-FREE
VEGETARIAN

Make Ahead Tip: Make this recipe ahead of time, then store in an airtight container and refrigerate for up to 2 days.

1. In a large bowl, whisk together the yogurt, chutney, and curry powder. Season with salt and pepper. Stir in the crumbled tofu, celery, grapes, apple, and onion.

2. Enjoy on a bed of romaine lettuce or in your favorite gluten-free wrap with romaine lettuce for crunch.

Per Serving: Calories: 235; Total Fat: 8g; Saturated Fat: 2g; Carbohydrates: 25g; Fiber: 4g; Sugar: 18g; Protein: 21g; Iron: 4mg; Sodium: 79mg

Ginger Veggie Stir-Fry

Prep time: 10 minutes / *Cook time:* 15 minutes

Crispy tofu and fresh vegetables sautéed in a quick and easy garlic-sesame sauce makes for a great weeknight meal. This dish can be made with a wide variety of your favorite vegetables.

3 tablespoon sesame oil or vegetable oil

2 (14-ounce) packages extra-firm tofu, drained, pressed, and cut into ¾-inch cubes

3 tablespoons tamari, divided

½ cup finely chopped onion

2 tablespoons minced garlic

1 tablespoon minced and peeled fresh ginger or 1 teaspoon ground ginger

1 to 2 teaspoons fresh chili paste or ¼ to ½ teaspoon red pepper flakes

1 cup chopped fresh broccoli florets

½ cup shredded carrots

½ cup chopped red bell pepper

½ cup chopped green bell pepper

½ cup fresh sugar snap peas

MAKES 4 SERVINGS

30-MINUTE
DAIRY-FREE
NUT-FREE
EGG-FREE
VEGAN

Allergen Tip: If you cannot tolerate soy, consider swapping out the tamari for Bragg Liquid Aminos and use chicken or shrimp instead of tofu.

Per Serving: Calories: 165; Total Fat: 13g; Saturated Fat: 2g; Carbohydrates: 7g; Fiber: 2g; Sugar: 3g; Protein: 7g; Iron: 2mg; Sodium: 776mg

1. In a large nonstick skillet or wok, heat the oil over medium-high heat. Once hot, add the tofu and 1 tablespoon tamari. Sauté, stirring occasionally, until the tofu is lightly colored, about 8 minutes. Add the onion, garlic, ginger, chili paste, and the remaining 2 tablespoons tamari. Stir and cook until fragrant, about 1 minute.

2. Add the broccoli, carrots, bell peppers, and peas. Sauté for 5 to 8 minutes, until cooked but still crisp.

3. Serve hot, with your preferred grain—brown rice, quinoa, gluten-free noodles, or cauliflower rice—along with additional tamari to taste.

Chickpea-Broccoli au Gratin

Prep time: 15 minutes / *Cook time:* 25 minutes

This vegetarian casserole is such a hearty meal, you won't miss the meat! Crisp broccoli combines with creamy quinoa and a zing of sun-dried tomatoes for an irresistible meal.

2 (15-ounce) cans chickpeas, drained and rinsed

2 cups cooked quinoa

2 cups broccoli florets (fresh or frozen)

2 cups shredded sharp cheddar cheese, divided

1 cup low-fat milk

⅓ cup chopped red onion

3 tablespoons chopped sun-dried tomatoes (optional)

1 tablespoon minced garlic

Salt

Freshly ground black pepper

½ cup gluten-free breadcrumbs

SERVES 4

EGG-FREE
NUT-FREE
VEGETARIAN

Ingredient Tip: When gluten-free bread gets old, you can save money by turning it into breadcrumbs instead of tossing it. Simply tear up the bread, place it in a food processor, and pulse until you have the size you're looking for. Add salt and seasonings that you enjoy and toast in an oven at 375°F for 5 to 8 minutes, stirring midway, until crisp.

1. Preheat the oven to 400°F. Grease a 9-by-9-inch baking dish.

2. In a large bowl, combine the chickpeas, quinoa, broccoli, 1 cup of cheese, milk, onion, sun-dried tomatoes (if using), and garlic. Season with salt and pepper.

3. Pour into the baking dish. Top with the remaining 1 cup of cheese and sprinkle with breadcrumbs.

4. Bake, uncovered, for 25 minutes, until the top is golden. Allow to cool for 10 minutes before serving.

Ingredient Tip: Getting enough iron can be tricky for those forgoing meat. Pairing them with a food high in vitamin C such as tomatoes enhances iron absorption.

Per Serving: Calories: 472; Total Fat: 14g; Saturated Fat: 6g; Carbohydrates: 66g; Fiber: 10g; Sugar: 2g; Protein: 21g; Iron: 3mg; Sodium: 744mg

Baked Cauliflower Mac 'n' Cheese

Prep time: 15 minutes / *Cook time:* 40 minutes

This is a rich, filling, one-pan meal. It provides a balance of protein, carbohydrates, and fat while boasting more iron than any meat-based dish.

2 tablespoons extra-virgin olive oil

½ cup chopped celery

⅓ onion, chopped

1 tablespoon minced garlic

1 cauliflower head, chopped

2 cups gluten-free pasta, cooked al dente (such as Banza)

1 (15-ounce) can chickpeas, drained and rinsed

1 (12-ounce) can gluten-free cream of celery soup (such as Pacific Foods)

½ cup sour cream or cream cheese

½ cup whole milk

1 cup shredded sharp cheddar cheese, divided

½ cup gluten-free breadcrumbs

SERVES 6

EGG-FREE
NUT-FREE
VEGETARIAN

Ingredient Tip:
Cauliflower is a fantastic addition to any mac 'n' cheese dish. It has a neutral flavor but adds volume and fiber, as well as a variety of B vitamins.

Per Serving: Calories: 442;
Total Fat: 21g;
Saturated Fat: 8g;
Carbohydrates: 48g;
Fiber: 10g; Sugar: 6g;
Protein: 20g; Iron: 5mg;
Sodium: 800mg

1. Preheat the oven to 400°F. Lightly oil an 8-inch square baking dish.

2. In a medium sauté pan or skillet, heat the olive oil over medium-high heat. Add the celery, onion, and garlic and cook for about 3 minutes, until fragrant.

3. In a large bowl, combine the cauliflower, pasta, chickpeas, soup, sour cream, milk, and ½ cup of cheddar cheese. Add the sautéed vegetables and mix well.

4. Pour the mixture into the prepared baking dish. Top with remaining ½ cup of cheese. Sprinkle with breadcrumbs.

5. Bake for 35 to 40 minutes, uncovered, until golden brown.

Simple Spaghetti Squash Bake

Prep time: 15 minutes / *Cook time:* 50 minutes

Spaghetti squash is a great gluten-free, low-carb alternative to pasta. It has a neutral flavor that allows for a variety of flavors, ranging from this traditional red sauce dish to a pesto festivity. It's best paired with a protein source, such as ground turkey, grilled chicken, or tempeh.

1 spaghetti squash

½ cup water

2 tablespoons extra-virgin olive oil

½ red bell pepper, chopped

½ green bell pepper, chopped

⅓ red onion, chopped

2 tablespoons minced garlic

1 (32-ounce) can crushed tomatoes

¼ cup chopped fresh basil or 2 tablespoons dried basil

Salt

Freshly ground black pepper

1 cup ricotta cheese

1 cup shredded mozzarella

SERVES 6

EGG-FREE
NUT-FREE
VEGETARIAN

Substitution Tip: This recipe allows you to make your own tomato sauce. To make this dish in a fraction of the time (and effort), use your favorite canned spaghetti sauce.

1. Preheat the oven to 400°F.

2. Carefully remove the ends of a spaghetti squash and cut in half lengthwise. Place in a microwave-safe bowl with the water. Microwave for 20 minutes, or until soft. Carefully remove from the microwave and let stand until cool enough to handle. Remove the seeds. Scoop the flesh from the shell and place in an 8-inch square baking dish.

3. In a sauté pan or skillet, heat the olive oil over medium-high heat. Sauté the peppers, onion, and garlic. Cook until fragrant, about 3 minutes. Add the tomatoes and basil and season with salt and pepper. Simmer for about 15 minutes, until slightly reduced and thickened.

4. Pour the tomato mixture over the spaghetti squash. Layer the ricotta cheese and mozzarella over top.

5. Bake for 35 minutes, until golden.

Per Serving: Calories: 135; Total Fat: 9g; Saturated Fat: 3g; Carbohydrates: 7g; Fiber: 1g; Sugar: 2g; Protein: 7g; Iron: 1mg; Sodium: 116mg

Ricotta-Stuffed Zucchini with Tempeh

Prep time: 15 minutes / *Cook time:* 25 minutes

Make the most of the zucchini harvest with this creamy vegetarian entrée. Zucchini boats pair well with Italian flavors, whether you're using a tomato sauce or a creamy ricotta atop the protein-rich tempeh.

2 tablespoons extra-virgin olive oil, divided

1 (8-ounce) block tempeh, crumbled

¼ cup chopped onion

2 tablespoons minced garlic

¼ teaspoon salt

4 small zucchinis

1 cup ricotta cheese

4 tablespoons grated Parmesan cheese, divided

1 tablespoon freshly squeezed lemon juice

1 cup halved cherry tomatoes

SERVES 4

EGG-FREE
NUT-FREE
VEGETARIAN

Ingredient Tip: Tempeh is made from fermented, pressed soybeans. The fermentation process creates a hearty dose of probiotics and makes the beans easier to digest. Some tempeh brands might include other grains—such as brown rice, millet, and other seeds—but many brands are gluten-free and even pasteurized.

1. In a large nonstick sauté pan or skillet, heat 1 tablespoon olive oil over medium-high heat. Add the crumbled tempeh, onion, garlic, and salt. Lightly sauté until the tempeh is brown and the mixture is fragrant, 3 to 5 minutes. Remove from the heat.

2. Preheat the oven to 475°F and place a small rimmed baking sheet in the oven as it heats.

3. Cut the zucchinis in half lengthwise and, using a spoon, remove the seeds and discard. Then remove about half of the zucchini flesh and set aside. Brush the cut sides of the zucchinis with the remaining 1 tablespoon oil, then place on the heated baking sheet, cut-side down. Roast for 10 minutes.

4. Meanwhile, mix together the ricotta, 2 tablespoons Parmesan cheese, lemon juice, and zucchini flesh.

5. Divide the tempeh mixture between the shells and then divide the ricotta mixture on top. Top with cherry tomatoes and remaining 2 tablespoons Parmesan cheese.

6. Broil until the tops are beginning to brown, 3 to 5 minutes.

Per Serving: Calories: 304; Total Fat: 20g; Saturated Fat: 6g; Carbohydrates: 16g; Fiber: 2g; Sugar: 3g; Protein: 22g; Iron: 2mg; Sodium: 310mg

Hearty Mexican-Style Skillet

Prep time: 8 minutes / *Cook time:* 8 minutes

This meal bursts with flavor in a few short minutes. Enjoy it on rice, quinoa, a bed of lettuce, or your favorite gluten-free wrap along with salsa and avocado. If you're avoiding dairy, simply don't add the cheese.

3 tablespoons extra-virgin olive oil

½ green bell pepper, chopped

½ red bell pepper, chopped

⅓ red onion, chopped

1 tablespoon minced garlic

1 (15-ounce) can black beans, drained and rinsed

1 cup chopped fresh spinach

½ cup corn, fresh or frozen

½ cup halved cherry tomatoes

1 teaspoon chili powder

1 teaspoon paprika

1 teaspoon ancho chili powder

Salt

Freshly ground black pepper

2 cups cooked rice

½ cup salsa, for serving

1 avocado, pitted, peeled, and chopped, for serving

4 ounces tortilla chips, for serving

½ cup shredded cheddar cheese, for serving

SERVES 4

30-MINUTE
EGG-FREE
NUT-FREE
VEGETARIAN

Ingredient Tip: Black beans are a nutritious staple for anyone trying to limit meat in their diet, as they are high in protein and iron. Pairing with a vitamin C–rich food such as tomatoes makes it easier for the body to absorb the iron in the beans.

1. In a large sauté pan or skillet, heat the olive oil over medium-high heat. Add the bell peppers, onion, and garlic. Sauté until fragrant, about 3 minutes. Add the black beans, spinach, corn, tomatoes, chili powder, paprika, and ancho chili powder. Season with salt and pepper and sauté for about 5 minutes, until cooked but still crisp.

2. Serve over rice with desired toppings.

Per Serving: Calories: 532; Total Fat: 24g; Saturated Fat: 6g; Carbohydrates: 68g; Fiber: 13g; Sugar: 4g; Protein: 16g; Iron: 10mg; Sodium: 311mg

15-Minute Chickpea Skillet

Prep time: 10 minutes / *Cook time:* 10 minutes

This colorful dish is similar to a lemon chicken without the chicken. It's full of flavor and ready in less than 20 minutes.

3 tablespoons
    extra-virgin olive oil

½ green bell pepper,
    chopped

½ red bell pepper,
    chopped

½ cup peeled,
    chopped carrots

⅓ red onion, chopped

1 tablespoon
    minced garlic

1 (15-ounce) can
    chickpeas, drained
    and rinsed

1 cup chopped
    fresh spinach

3 tablespoons chopped
    sun-dried tomatoes

2 tablespoons freshly
    squeezed lemon juice

1 tablespoon
    chopped capers

⅓ cup shredded
    Parmesan cheese

2 cups cooked
    gluten-free pasta
    (such as Banza),
    for serving

SERVES 4

30-MINUTE
EGG-FREE
NUT-FREE
VEGETARIAN

Substitution Tip: To make this dish dairy-free or vegan, swap the Parmesan cheese for nutritional yeast.

1. In a large sauté pan or skillet, heat the olive oil over medium-high heat. Add the bell peppers, carrots, onion, and garlic and sauté for 3 to 5 minutes, until the carrots are slightly soft. Add the chickpeas, spinach, sun-dried tomatoes, lemon juice, and capers. Sauté another 5 minutes. Mix in the Parmesan cheese.

2. Serve over pasta.

Per Serving: Calories: 466; Total Fat: 18g; Saturated Fat: 3g; Carbohydrates: 60g; Fiber: 15g; Sugar: 12g; Protein: 24g; Iron: 8mg; Sodium: 241mg

Coconut-Chickpea Curry

Prep time: 5 minutes / *Cook time:* 20 minutes

A classic curry inspired by Indian flavors, this chickpea curry skips the complicated steps but doesn't skimp on flavor.

1 tablespoon
    vegetable oil

½ red onion, chopped

3 tablespoons
    minced garlic

1 tablespoon minced
    and peeled fresh
    ginger or 1 teaspoon
    ground ginger

¼ teaspoon
    ground turmeric

¼ teaspoon ground
    cayenne pepper

Salt

Freshly ground
    black pepper

1 (14.5-ounce) can diced
    tomatoes, drained

1 (15-ounce) can
    chickpeas, drained
    and rinsed

1 (13.5-ounce) can full-fat
    coconut milk

2 cups cooked rice

SERVES 4

30-MINUTE
DAIRY-FREE
EGG-FREE
NUT-FREE
VEGAN

Substitution Tip:
Experiment with your favorite vegetables in this dish, such as bell peppers, carrots, sweet potato, eggplant, and zucchini.

1. In a large sauté pan or skillet, heat the oil over medium-high heat. Add the red onion and garlic. Cook for about 3 minutes, until fragrant.

2. Reduce the heat to medium. Add the ginger, turmeric, and cayenne pepper and season with salt and pepper. Add the tomatoes to the pan and stir well. Continue to cook, stirring occasionally, for 3 to 5 minutes. Stir in the chickpeas and coconut milk. Bring the mixture to a boil, then reduce the heat to medium-low.

3. Simmer the coconut-chickpea curry for about 10 minutes, or until reduced slightly. Season with salt and pepper. Serve over rice.

Per Serving: Calories: 290; Total Fat: 6g; Saturated Fat: 2g; Carbohydrates: 50g; Fiber: 5g; Sugar: 3g; Protein: 8g; Iron: 3mg; Sodium: 367mg

Butternut Squash Quesadilla

Prep time: 5 minutes / *Cook time:* 6 to 8 minutes

Quesadillas go from refrigerator to table in minutes. The addition of chickpeas and vegetables enhances the nutrients of this favorite. Consider adding avocado or dipping in salsa for more flavor.

½ cup cooked, mashed butternut squash, divided

4 (7-inch) gluten-free tortillas

½ cup chickpeas, divided

⅓ cup halved cherry tomatoes, divided

¼ cup chopped red onion, divided

1 teaspoon garlic powder, divided

½ cup shredded mozzarella cheese, divided

SERVES 2

30-MINUTE
EGG-FREE
NUT-FREE
VEGETARIAN

Ingredient Tip: For more protein, crumble and lightly sauté tempeh in vegetable oil. Season with a sprinkle of garlic, chili powder, salt, and pepper.

1. Heat a sauté pan or skillet over medium-high heat.

2. Spread half of the butternut squash over 1 tortilla. Layer with half of the chickpeas, tomatoes, onion, garlic powder, and mozzarella cheese. Cover with another tortilla.

3. Carefully transfer to the hot skillet. Heat for 2 to 3 minutes. Carefully flip and heat another 2 to 3 minutes.

4. Repeat with the remaining ingredients.

Per Serving: Calories: 258; Total Fat: 6g; Saturated Fat: 2g; Carbohydrates: 45g; Fiber: 7g; Sugar: 4g; Protein: 8g; Iron: 3mg; Sodium: 636mg

Rainbow Grain Bowl

Prep time: 15 minutes

This dish features beautiful layers of color and flavor from a nourishing combination of vegetables, nuts, grains, and seeds. Enjoy with Greek Yogurt Ranch Dip (page 106) or your favorite store-bought ranch dressing.

2 cups cooked
   quinoa or rice

2 cups cooked chickpeas
   or lentils

1½ cups corn kernels
   (fresh, thawed from
   frozen, or rinsed
   from a can)

1½ cups sliced
   cherry tomatoes

1½ cups sliced
   cucumbers

1½ cups snap peas

2 avocados, halved,
   pitted, and sliced

¾ cup chopped
   fresh basil

6 tablespoons nuts or
   seeds (sesame seeds,
   pumpkin seeds,
   almonds, cashews,
   or pecans)

2 tablespoons
   garlic powder

¾ cup Greek Yogurt
   Ranch Dip (page 106),
   for serving

SERVES 6

**30-MINUTE
EGG-FREE
VEGETARIAN**

Prep Ahead Tip: Grain bowls are great to assemble in advance because none of the vegetables get soggy like a traditional salad. Simply assemble in airtight containers and store in the refrigerator for 3 to 5 days for easy grab-and-go meals. For best results, keep the avocado and ranch separate until ready to serve.

In six bowls, divide the quinoa, chickpeas, corn, tomatoes, cucumbers, and peas. Add a few avocado slices, sprinkle with basil, nuts, and garlic powder, and drizzle with ranch dressing.

Per Serving: Calories: 380; Total Fat: 16g; Saturated Fat: 3g; Carbohydrates: 52g; Fiber: 13g; Sugar: 5g; Protein: 12g; Iron: 3mg; Sodium: 258mg

Real Talk About Celiac

"I try to pack my meals for the week each weekend. But when I travel, there's no time before going back to real life on Mondays. For those times, I make sure to stock up on gluten-free frozen meals and soups that I can pair with some fresh or frozen vegetables."

Barbecue-Ready Black Bean Burger

Prep time: 5 minutes / *Cook time:* 8 minutes

Veggie burgers are a fantastic addition to any barbecue, but many are too fragile to be grilled. This hearty burger can withstand the rigor of the grill and is delicious to boot. Enjoy with your favorite burger fixings or placed on top of a salad.

1 cup cashews or gluten-free breadcrumbs

½ red onion, finely chopped

2 tablespoons minced garlic

1 tablespoon chili powder

1 tablespoon ground cumin

1 tablespoon paprika

Salt

Freshly ground black pepper

1 cup cooked brown rice or quinoa

1 (15-ounce) can black beans, drained and rinsed

⅓ cup gluten-free breadcrumbs

¼ cup barbecue sauce

SERVES 6

30-MINUTE
DAIRY-FREE
EGG-FREE
VEGAN

Make Ahead Tip: To freeze for later, cook the burgers as instructed. Once cool, place in an airtight bag or container and freeze for up to 3 weeks. For a crisp finish, reheat in a 400°F oven until warmed through, about 15 minutes. For a softer finish, microwave for 1 to 2 minutes.

1. Heat a grill to medium-high heat. Oil the grill grates.

2. In a food processor or blender, pulse the cashews, onion, garlic, chili powder, cumin, paprika, salt, and pepper until roughly chopped. Transfer to a bowl and mash with the rice, black beans, breadcrumbs, and barbecue sauce.

3. Form the mixture into 6 patties, ¾-inch thick.

4. Grill for 8 minutes, gently flipping halfway through.

Per Serving: Calories: 360; Total Fat: 12g; Saturated Fat: 2g; Carbohydrates: 53g; Fiber: 7g; Sugar: 4g; Protein: 12g; Iron: 3mg; Sodium: 272mg

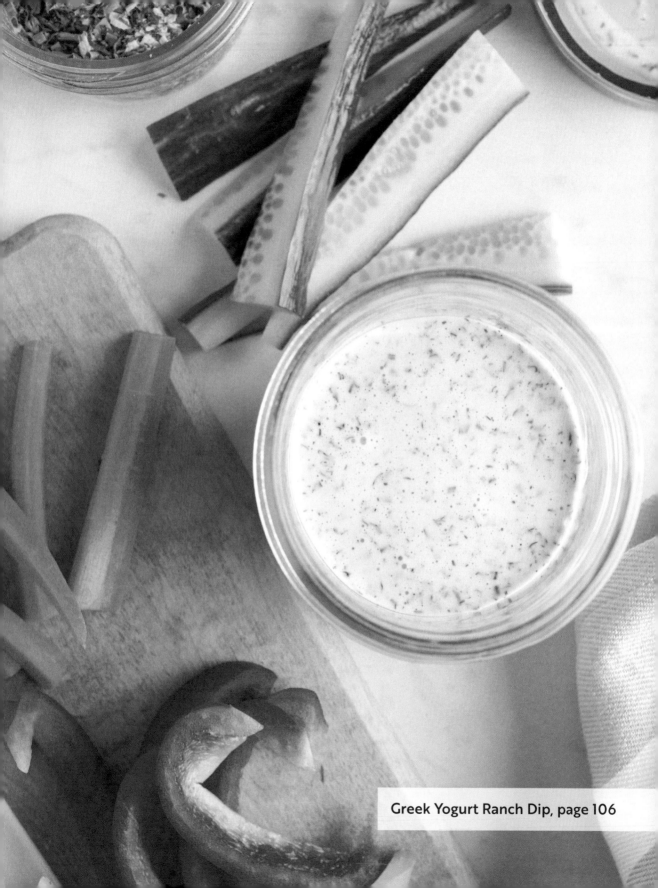

Greek Yogurt Ranch Dip, page 106

Sides and Snacks

Greek Yogurt Ranch Dip

Prep time: 10 minutes

Greek yogurt dips are a delicious, heart-healthy alternative to ranch dressings and vegetable dips. Pair this dish with your favorite raw vegetables or gluten-free chips.

2 cups plain
  Greek yogurt

½ cup grated
  Parmesan cheese

1 tablespoon
  minced garlic

1 teaspoon dry chives

3 to 4 tablespoons
  freshly squeezed
  lemon juice

Salt

Freshly ground
  black pepper

MAKES ABOUT
2½ CUPS

30-MINUTE

EGG-FREE

NUT-FREE

VEGETARIAN

In a bowl, combine the yogurt, Parmesan cheese, garlic, chives, and lemon juice and mix well. Season with salt and pepper. Serve.

Per Serving (⅓ cup): Calories: 63; Total Fat: 3g; Saturated Fat: 2g; Carbohydrates: 3g; Fiber: 0g; Sugar: 2g; Protein: 8g; Iron: 0mg; Sodium: 83mg

Ingredient Tip:
Traditional ranch dressing is made with oil, egg yolk, and other flavorings. By using Greek yogurt, you get the same rich, milky consistency of ranch without the higher saturated fat and calorie content.

Green Goddess Dip

Prep time: 10 minutes

If you're looking to bulk up your guacamole with protein and fiber, look no further than this spin on an old classic. After you've made the dip, bust out your favorite gluten-free tortilla chips and enjoy your hard work.

1 (15-ounce) can chickpeas, drained and rinsed or 1½ cup cooked chickpeas

1 avocado, halved, pitted, and peeled

½ cup fresh cilantro leaves

⅓ medium red onion

¼ cup freshly squeezed lemon juice

¼ cup extra-virgin olive oil

2 garlic cloves, peeled

½ teaspoon chili powder

½ cup chopped tomatoes

Salt

Freshly ground black pepper

MAKES ABOUT 2½ CUPS

30-MINUTE
DAIRY-FREE
EGG-FREE
NUT-FREE
VEGAN

In a food processor or blender, combine the chickpeas, avocado, cilantro, onion, lemon juice, olive oil, garlic, and chili powder and blend until smooth. Pour into a serving dish and top with the tomatoes. Season with salt and pepper. Serve.

Per Serving (⅓ cup): Calories: 143; Total Fat: 12g; Saturated Fat: 2g; Carbohydrates: 8g; Fiber: 3g; Sugar: 1g; Protein: 3g; Iron: 1mg; Sodium: 54mg

Ingredient Tip: Note that avocados can turn brown when exposed to air. Eating browned avocado will not harm anyone, but it's less visually appealing. To reduce this, make sure to store your avocado in an airtight container in the refrigerator. Additionally, using lemon and tomato in this recipe provides vitamin C, which can protect the avocado from browning.

Sun-Dried Tomato-Basil Hummus

Prep time: 10 minutes

Hummus is perhaps the quickest nutrition-packed snack possible. This recipe has fresh notes inspired by Italian flavors. Use it as an appetizer with raw vegetables or your favorite gluten-free crackers, or as an alternative to mayonnaise on a gluten-free sandwich.

1 (15-ounce) can chickpeas, drained and rinsed or 1½ cups cooked chickpeas

⅓ medium red onion

⅓ cup fresh basil leaves

¼ cup sun-dried tomatoes

¼ cup extra-virgin olive oil

1 garlic clove, peeled

Salt

Freshly ground black pepper

MAKES ABOUT 2 CUPS

30-MINUTE
DAIRY-FREE
EGG-FREE
NUT-FREE
VEGAN

In a food processor or blender, combine the chickpeas, onion, basil, tomatoes, olive oil, and garlic and blend until smooth. Season with salt and pepper. Serve.

Per Serving (⅓ cup): Calories: 149; Total Fat: 9g; Saturated Fat: 1g; Carbohydrates: 15g; Fiber: 3g; Sugar: 5g; Protein: 3g; Iron: 1mg; Sodium: 227mg

Substitution Tip: The magic of hummus is how simple and versatile it is. Another popular variation is "everything" hummus. Simply follow the same directions but instead of tomatoes and basil, add 2 tablespoons of "everything but the bagel" seasoning. (Available at most grocery stores, this is a combination of sesame seeds, poppy seeds, garlic, and onion.)

No-Cook Spinach-Artichoke Dip

Prep time: 10 minutes

Whether you're hosting a gathering at your home or looking for a delicious appetizer, this no-cook dip is a nourishing addition with great flavor and a healthy serving of iron, protein, and fiber. Enjoy with your favorite raw vegetables and gluten-free chips.

1 (15-ounce) can chickpeas, drained and rinsed

1 (10-ounce) package frozen chopped spinach, thawed, drained, and chopped

1 cup grated or shredded Parmesan cheese

1 (8-ounce) package reduced-fat cream cheese, softened

1 cup plain Greek yogurt

½ red onion, chopped

3 tablespoons minced garlic

1 (14-ounce) can artichoke hearts, drained and chopped

MAKES ABOUT 6 CUPS

30-MINUTE

EGG-FREE

NUT-FREE

VEGETARIAN

Substitution Tip: To make this dish dairy free, use 1½ cups soaked cashews and 1 cup plant-based milk in place of the cream cheese and yogurt. Use nutritional yeast instead of Parmesan cheese to enhance the flavor as well as get a boost of vitamin B12.

In a food processor, blend together the chickpeas, spinach, Parmesan cheese, cream cheese, yogurt, onion, and garlic. Process until smooth. Add the artichoke hearts and lightly pulse. Serve.

Per Serving (1 cup): Calories: 172; Total Fat: 7g; Saturated Fat: 4g; Carbohydrates: 15g; Fiber: 5g; Sugar: 3g; Protein: 13g; Iron: 2mg; Sodium: 621mg

Avocado-Black Bean Dip

Prep time: 10 minutes

This dip is the definition of heart-healthy, boasting high levels of fiber and anti-oxidants. Enjoy it along with your favorite gluten-free crackers or make it into a meal by serving with a side of rice and your favorite protein.

1 (15-ounce) can black beans, drained and rinsed

1 avocado, peeled, pitted, and mashed

1 tablespoon freshly squeezed lime juice

1 tablespoon minced garlic

Salt

Freshly ground black pepper

2 medium tomatoes, chopped

¼ cup chopped red onion

MAKES ABOUT 3 CUPS

30-MINUTE
DAIRY-FREE
EGG-FREE
NUT-FREE
VEGAN

In a bowl, mash the black beans, avocado, lime juice, and garlic together. Season with salt and pepper and top with the tomatoes and onion. Serve.

Per Serving (½ cup): Calories: 127; Total Fat: 7g; Saturated Fat: 2g; Carbohydrates: 13g; Fiber: 6g; Sugar: 1g; Protein: 5g; Iron: 1mg; Sodium: 101mg

Ingredient Tip: Tomatoes are high in nutrients called antioxidants and carotenoids that protect the body from cellular damage. When tomatoes are eaten along with healthier fats, like avocado, the body absorbs more of the tomato's phytochemicals.

Roasted Zucchini with Parmesan

Prep time: 10 minutes / *Cook time:* 15 minutes

Zucchini is a versatile vegetable that cooks in an instant. This dish is a fantastic side for grilled chicken or beef along with a starch, like a baked potato. It's a perfect complement to Grilled Spicy Salmon with Rub (page 71).

4 medium zucchinis and/or yellow summer squash, cut into ½-inch-thick rounds

½ cup sliced onion

⅓ cup grated Parmesan cheese, divided

1 tablespoon extra-virgin olive oil

½ teaspoon salt

¼ teaspoon freshly ground black pepper

SERVES 4

30-MINUTE
EGG-FREE
NUT-FREE
VEGETARIAN

1. Preheat the oven to 450°F. Line a baking sheet with parchment paper or lightly oil.

2. In a large bowl, combine the zucchinis, onion, half the Parmesan cheese, olive oil, salt, and pepper.

3. Roast in the oven until the zucchini is just cooked through and beginning to brown, 10 to 15 minutes. Sprinkle with the remaining Parmesan. Enjoy immediately.

Per Serving: Calories: 112; Total Fat: 7g; Saturated Fat: 3g; Carbohydrates: 8g; Fiber: 3g; Sugar: 4g; Protein: 7g; Iron: 1mg; Sodium: 441mg

Ingredient Tip: While zucchini is considered a vegetable by many, it's botanically classified as a fruit. It is rich in many nutrients but particularly high in vitamin A, with 1 cup providing 40 percent of your daily requirement, supporting vision and the immune system.

Substitution Tip: Make this recipe vegan by substituting the Parmesan cheese with nutritional yeast.

Lemon Roasted Mixed Vegetables

Prep time: 10 minutes / *Cook time:* 25 minutes

Roasting vegetables with lemon not only improves the absorption of iron, but it also gives a bright flavor to a warm classic.

1½ cups cauliflower florets

1½ cups broccoli florets

2 tablespoons minced garlic

2 tablespoons extra-virgin olive oil

1 teaspoon dried crushed oregano

¼ teaspoon salt

1 red bell pepper, cut into 1-inch chunks

1 zucchini, cut into 1-inch-thick slices

½ cup freshly squeezed lemon juice

SERVES 6

DAIRY-FREE
EGG-FREE
NUT-FREE
VEGAN

Ingredient Tip: Broccoli and cauliflower are part of the cruciferous vegetable family. Cruciferous vegetables are good sources of various phytonutrients, which are plant-based compounds that may help lower inflammation and reduce the risk of developing cancer.

1. Preheat the oven to 425°F. Line a baking sheet with parchment paper.

2. On the baking sheet, combine the cauliflower, broccoli, and garlic and drizzle with oil. Sprinkle with oregano and salt. Roast for 10 minutes.

3. Add the bell pepper and zucchini to the pan and drizzle with lemon juice. Roast until the vegetables are crisp-tender and lightly browned, about 15 more minutes.

Per Serving: Calories: 112; Total Fat: 5g; Saturated Fat: 1g; Carbohydrates: 15g; Fiber: 5g; Sugar: 6g; Protein: 5g; Iron: 1mg; Sodium: 160mg

Roasted Edamame

Prep time: 5 minutes / *Cook time:* 15 minutes

Snacks that are convenient, satisfying, and nourishing aren't easily found in the grocery store. Roasted edamame is a perfect solution.

1 (16-ounce) bag frozen
    shelled edamame

3 tablespoons grated
    Parmesan cheese

Salt

Freshly ground
    black pepper

Red pepper
    flakes (optional)

1 tablespoon extra-virgin
    olive oil

SERVES 4

30-MINUTE
EGG-FREE
NUT-FREE
VEGETARIAN

1. Preheat the oven to 400°F. Line a baking sheet with parchment paper.

2. Pour the edamame on the baking sheet and season with the Parmesan, salt, pepper, and red pepper flakes (if using). Drizzle with olive oil and toss until evenly combined.

3. Bake for about 15 minutes, or until the edamame is crispy.

Per Serving: Calories:113; Total Fat: 7g; Saturated Fat: 2g; Carbohydrates: 5g; Fiber: 2g; Sugar: 1g; Protein: 7g; Iron: 1mg; Sodium: 70mg

Ingredient Tip: Edamame, or soybeans, are an excellent source of lean protein. Similar to other beans, 1 cup of edamame boasts 17 grams of satisfying protein and 8 grams of fiber, with 50 percent fewer grams of carbohydrates compared to black beans.

Spicy Roasted Chickpeas

Prep time: 5 minutes / *Cook time:* 30 minutes

Roasted chickpeas are a great alternative to nuts to enjoy alone as a snack or on top of a dish such as a salad.

1 (15-ounce) can chickpeas, rinsed or 1½ cup cooked chickpeas

1 tablespoon extra-virgin olive oil

2 teaspoons ground cumin

¼ teaspoon ground cayenne pepper

¼ teaspoon salt

SERVES 4

DAIRY-FREE
EGG-FREE
NUT-FREE
VEGAN

Make Ahead Tip: Once cooled, store these chickpeas without a sealed lid to maintain their crisp texture for up to 2 days.

1. Preheat the oven to 450°F and position the rack in the upper third of the oven.

2. Blot the chickpeas dry and toss in a bowl with the olive oil, cumin, cayenne, and salt. Spread on a rimmed baking sheet. Bake, stirring once or twice, until browned and crunchy, 25 to 30 minutes. Let cool on the baking sheet for 15 minutes before serving or storing.

Per Serving: Calories: 123; Total Fat: 5g; Saturated Fat: 5g; Carbohydrates: 17g; Fiber: 3g; Sugar: 0g; Protein: 4g; Iron: 2mg; Sodium: 373mg

Honey Roasted Curried Carrots

Prep time: 5 minutes / *Cook time:* 30 minutes

This Indian-inspired dish is a delicious spin on roasted vegetables. The curry pairs with the sweetness of the carrot to make a dish that can't be beat.

6 whole carrots, peeled and cut into ¼-inch-thick coins

2 tablespoons butter, melted

2 tablespoons honey

1 tablespoon curry powder

Salt

Freshly ground black pepper

SERVES 4

EGG-FREE
NUT-FREE
VEGETARIAN

1. Preheat the oven to 400°F.

2. Place the carrots in a small casserole dish or baking dish.

3. In a small bowl, mix together the butter, honey, and curry powder and season with salt and pepper. Pour over and evenly coat the carrots.

4. Bake for 25 to 30 minutes, until tender. Enjoy!

Per Serving: Calories: 135; Total Fat: 6g; Saturated Fat: 4g; Carbohydrates: 20g; Fiber: 3g; Sugar: 16g; Protein: 2g; Iron: 0mg; Sodium: 100mg

Ingredient Tip: Curry powder is a generic term for a blend of spices commonly associated with Indian cuisine. It typically includes spices such as turmeric, red chiles, coriander seeds, black pepper, cumin seeds, fenugreek seeds, curry leaves, mustard seeds, cinnamon, cardamom, cloves, nutmeg, peppercorns, and bay leaves. Curry has been shown to have health benefits such as reducing inflammation and improving digestion.

Cauliflower Fried Rice

Prep time: 10 minutes / *Cook time:* 15 minutes

This healthy twist on take-out fried rice uses cauliflower as its base in place of the rice. Minced cauliflower has a neutral flavor that takes on a similar texture to rice, while adding a healthy dose of antioxidants and fiber. Although this dish has an Asian flair, minced cauliflower can be used as a base for many rice-based dishes.

1 cauliflower head, broken into florets

2 tablespoons tamari or liquid aminos

3 tablespoons sesame oil, divided

1 teaspoon ground ginger or 1 tablespoon grated peeled fresh ginger

3 large eggs, beaten

½ onion, chopped

1 tablespoon minced garlic

1 cup chopped broccoli florets

2 carrots, peeled and grated

½ cup frozen peas

SERVES 6

30-MINUTE
DAIRY-FREE
NUT-FREE
VEGETARIAN

Prep Ahead Tip: If you love cauliflower rice but don't like the preparation process, you can prepare it in advance. Once pulsed, store in an airtight container. It will last in the refrigerator for 4 days and in the freezer for 2 months.

1. In the bowl of a food processor, pulse the cauliflower until it resembles rice, 2 to 3 minutes, then set aside. If you do not have a food processor, use a large cutting board and finely chop the cauliflower. (Note: This will be messy.)

2. In a small bowl, whisk together the tamari, 1 tablespoon of sesame oil, and ginger and set aside.

3. In a medium sauté pan or skillet, heat 1 tablespoon of sesame oil over low heat. Add the eggs and scramble for about 5 minutes, until cooked through, then set aside.

4. In a large skillet or wok, heat the remaining 1 tablespoon of sesame oil over medium-high heat. Add the onion and garlic to the skillet and cook, stirring often, until the onions are translucent, 3 to 4 minutes. Stir in the broccoli, carrots, and peas and cook, stirring constantly, until the vegetables are tender, 3 to 4 minutes.

5. Stir in the cauliflower rice, eggs, and tamari mixture. Cook, stirring constantly, until heated through and the cauliflower is tender, 3 to 4 minutes. Serve immediately.

Per Serving: Calories: 137; Total Fat: 9g; Saturated Fat: 2g; Carbohydrates: 8g; Fiber: 3g; Sugar: 4g; Protein: 6g; Iron: 1mg; Sodium: 403mg

Gluten-Free Bread

Prep time: 15 minutes / *Cook time:* 45 minutes

Gluten is what defines traditional bread, as it provides the elasticity that gives bread its chewy texture. Without gluten, breads can be dry or stiff. This recipe uses a flour blend and xanthan gum to get as close to the real thing as possible, all at a fraction of the cost of store-bought brands. Be warned that gluten-free batter is more like muffin batter than traditional bread dough and that's why no kneading is required.

¼ cup warm water

3 tablespoons granulated sugar

2 teaspoons active dry yeast

3 cups King Arthur Gluten-Free All-Purpose Flour

1¼ teaspoons salt

1½ teaspoons xanthan gum

¾ cup warm milk

4 tablespoons butter, softened

3 large eggs

SERVES 6

NUT-FREE

VEGETARIAN

Make Ahead Tip: Homemade bread is always best hot out of the oven. Shelf life on homemade bread is limited and gluten-free bread is no different. After the first day, reheat or toast and enjoy.

1. In a small bowl, combine the warm water, sugar, and yeast. Let stand for 15 minutes.

2. In a large bowl, stand mixer, or food processor with a dough blade, combine the flour, salt, and xanthan gum. Add the yeast mixture and mix until combined.

3. Slowly add in the milk and butter while continuing to beat.

4. Beat in the eggs, one at a time. Once all the ingredients are incorporated, beat at high speed for 3 minutes until the mixture is smooth, scraping down the sides as needed.

5. Into a greased loaf pan, transfer the dough and press so that it is level in the pan.

6. Cover with greased plastic wrap or a clean wet towel. Set in a warm place and allow to rise for 45 to 60 minutes.

7. Preheat the oven to 350°F.

8. Transfer the bread to the oven and bake for 40 to 45 minutes, until golden brown. Remove from the oven, turn it out of the pan, and allow the loaf to cool on a rack.

Per Serving: Calories: 163; Total Fat: 4g; Saturated Fat: 2g; Carbohydrates: 26g; Fiber: 0g; Sugar: 3g; Protein: 4g; Iron: 1mg; Sodium: 221mg

Creamed Corn with Red Peppers

Prep time: 15 minutes / *Cook time:* 25 minutes

This creamy side dish pairs well with chicken or beef over a bed of rice. This spin on creamed corn replaces some of the cream cheese with yogurt to make it more heart-healthy without sacrificing flavor or texture.

2 tablespoons butter

1 cup chopped onion

2 red bell peppers, chopped

1 tablespoon minced garlic

4 cups fresh or frozen corn kernels, thawed

¼ cup low-sodium chicken broth

⅛ teaspoon red pepper flakes

½ cup low-fat cream cheese, cut into small chunks

½ cup plain Greek yogurt

SERVES 8

EGG-FREE
NUT-FREE

Ingredient Tip: Corn has several health benefits. Its high fiber content supports digestion, and it is a great source of B vitamins, as well as the minerals zinc, magnesium, copper, iron, and manganese. It's also a good source of carotenoids, which promote eye health.

1. In a sauté pan or skillet, melt the butter over medium heat. Add the onion, bell pepper, and garlic, cooking until fragrant, about 3 minutes.

2. Turn the heat to low. Add the corn, broth, and red pepper flakes. Fold in the cream cheese and yogurt.

3. Allow to simmer 20 minutes, until thickened. Serve immediately.

Per Serving: Calories: 117; Total Fat: 4g; Saturated Fat: 2g; Carbohydrates: 20g; Fiber: 3g; Sugar: 5g; Protein: 4g; Iron: 1mg; Sodium: 29mg

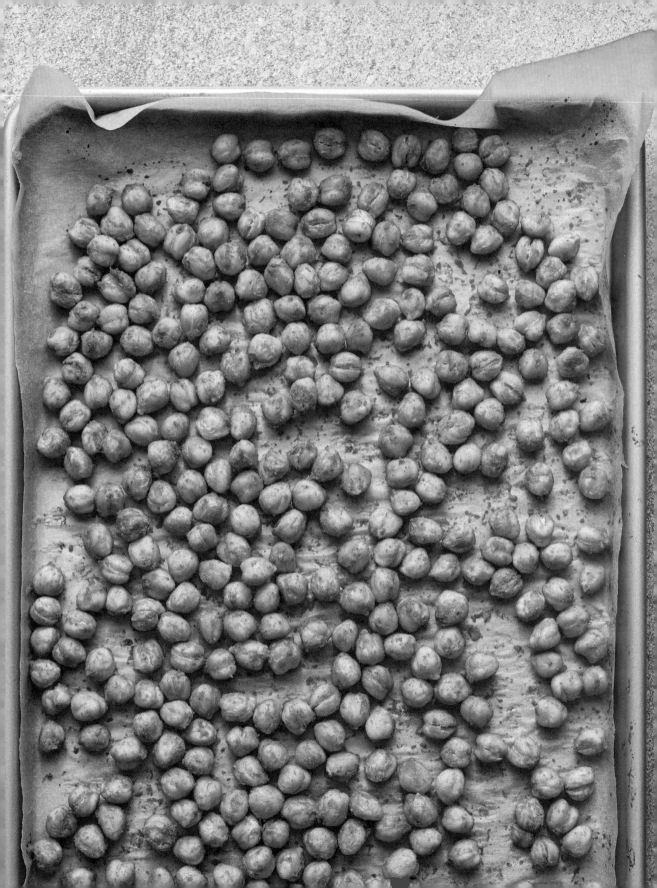

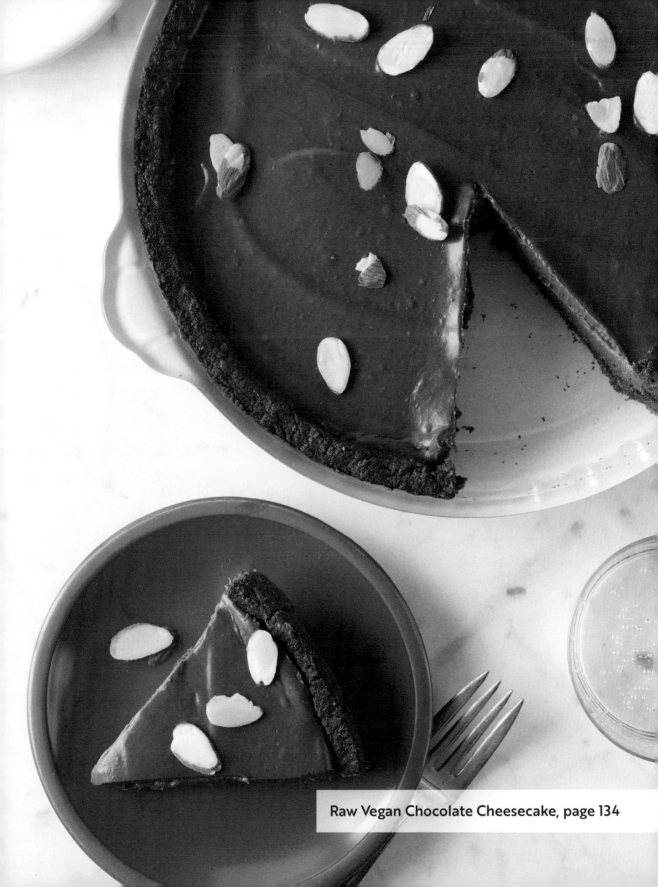

Raw Vegan Chocolate Cheesecake, page 134

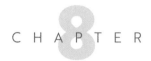

CHAPTER 8

Desserts

Fluffy Meringue Cookies

Prep time: 15 minutes / *Cook time:* 80 minutes

These meringue cookies are light and airy and just melt in your mouth. The outsides are nice and crisp, yet the insides remain wonderfully soft and puffy.

4 large egg whites

½ teaspoon vanilla extract (or other flavored extracts)

¼ teaspoon freshly squeezed lemon juice

¼ teaspoon salt

1 drop food coloring (optional)

¾ cup granulated sugar

MAKES 10 COOKIES

DAIRY-FREE

NUT-FREE

VEGETARIAN

Substitution Tip: For a variety of flavors, try adding almond extract, peppermint extract, or orange extract. You could even fold in freeze-dried fruit that's been ground.

1. Preheat the oven to 250°F. Line a baking sheet with parchment paper.

2. In a large mixing bowl, using a mixer on medium speed, whip the egg whites, vanilla, lemon juice, salt, and food coloring (if using) until foamy. Continue to whip and slowly add in the sugar, a spoonful at a time.

3. When all the sugar has been added, turn the mixer up to high speed and whip until the meringue is glossy and very stiff, 5 to 7 minutes.

4. For best visual results, use a clean piping bag with a French star tip to create 1-inch diameter kisses on parchment-lined sheet. But if you don't have a piping bag, use a spoon to create little 2-inch dollops of meringue.

5. Bake for 40 minutes, until firm to the touch. Once the baking time is completed, turn the oven off and leave the meringues inside, allowing them to continue to dry for another 60 minutes.

Per Serving (1 cookie): Calories: 63; Total Fat: 0g; Saturated Fat: 0g; Carbohydrates: 15g; Fiber: 0g; Sugar: 15g; Protein: 2g; Iron: 0mg; Sodium: 71mg

No-Bake Monster Cookies

Prep time: 10 minutes, plus 20 minutes to harden

These no-bake "cookies" are ready in less than 10 minutes. Whole grains and plant fats create energy that lasts and will satisfy any sweet tooth. To make this recipe oat-free, use gluten-free rice cereal instead of oats.

1½ cups rolled oats

½ cup peanut butter or sun butter

⅓ cup honey

¼ cup mini M&M's

¼ cup mini chocolate chips

¼ cup raisins or dry cranberries

1 teaspoon chia seeds or ground flaxseed (optional)

½ teaspoon vanilla extract

MAKES 16 COOKIES

30-MINUTE VEGETARIAN

Make Ahead Tip:
Store the leftovers in a resealable bag in the refrigerator for up to 5 days or in the freezer for up to 1 month.

1. In a medium bowl, combine the oats, peanut butter, honey, M&M's, chocolate chips, raisins, chia seeds (if using), and vanilla. Stir well until combined.

2. Line a baking sheet with parchment paper. Roll the dough into 1½-inch balls and set them on the baking sheet.

3. Refrigerate for 20 minutes, until hardened.

Per Serving (1 cookie): Calories: 115; Total Fat: 6g; Saturated Fat: 2g; Carbohydrates: 15g; Fiber: 1g; Sugar: 11g; Protein: 3g; Iron: 1mg; Sodium: 42mg

Cookie "Dough" Dip

Prep time: 5 minutes

This delicious recipe tastes just like raw cookie dough without the eggs or gluten. Serve with gluten-free cookies, graham crackers, or fresh fruit like strawberries. It's also a great addition to ice cream.

1 (15-ounce) can chickpeas or white beans, drained and rinsed

¼ cup nut butter (peanut butter, almond butter, or sun butter)

½ cup brown sugar

2 to 3 tablespoons ground flaxseed or chia seeds (optional)

2 teaspoons vanilla extract

⅛ teaspoon salt

⅓ cup chocolate chips

MAKES ABOUT 2½ CUPS

30-MINUTE

EGG-FREE

VEGETARIAN

In a food processor, combine the chickpeas, nut butter, brown sugar, flaxseed, vanilla, and salt. Mix well. Fold in the chocolate chips. Put in a serving bowl and enjoy!

Allergen Tip: Sun butter is made from sunflower seeds and a safe alternative for those with a tree nut or peanut allergy. Additionally, this recipe can be made without the nut butter.

Per Serving (⅓ cup): Calories: 173; Total Fat: 7g; Saturated Fat: 2g; Carbohydrates: 24g; Fiber: 3g; Sugar: 13g; Protein: 5g; Iron: 2mg; Sodium: 215mg

Mint-Chocolate Chip
Nice Cream

Prep time: 5 minutes

Not sure what to do with overripe bananas? Freeze them and enjoy some "nice" cream. The frozen bananas have a similar texture and flavor to ice cream without the dairy.

2 or 3 overripe, frozen
  bananas, peeled

⅛ teaspoon
  peppermint extract

Pinch salt

⅓ cup mini
  chocolate chips

SERVES 2

30-MINUTE
EGG-FREE
NUT-FREE
VEGETARIAN

In a food processor or blender, combine the frozen bananas, peppermint, and salt. Blend until creamy. Fold in the chocolate chips. Enjoy!

Per Serving: Calories: 215; Total Fat: 6g; Saturated Fat: 5g; Carbohydrates: 40g; Fiber: 3g; Sugar: 26g; Protein: 2g; Iron: 1mg; Sodium: 11mg

Substitution Tip: Get creative with the recipe and make your own variations. Use peanut butter and chocolate or add raspberries and avocado for a sweet treat.

Real Talk About Celiac

"Sometimes it's tempting to eat a bit of cake—I really missed the ease of my old food! But intentionally eating gluten not only caused physical harm, it also confused those around me. I used to intentionally eat bread when my friends wanted to grab a sandwich. But that sent the message that being gluten-free wasn't important and they pressured me more and more, saying, 'You ate it yesterday—what does it matter?'"

Rich Chocolate Chia Pudding

Prep time: 10 minutes, plus 3 hours to chill

The chia seeds in this pudding make it a nutritious option, boasting fiber and omega-3 fatty acids. Adding seasonal fruit right before you serve this dish adds color and is a great way to vary the recipe.

¼ cup unsweetened cocoa powder

3 tablespoons maple syrup

½ teaspoon vanilla extract

Pinch sea salt

1½ cups whole milk

½ cup chia seeds

SERVES 4

EGG-FREE
NUT-FREE
VEGETARIAN

1. In a small bowl, combine the cocoa, maple syrup, vanilla, and salt. Whisk well to combine. Add 2 tablespoons of milk to form a paste, before adding the remaining milk (this helps keep the cocoa powder from clumping).

2. Add the chia seeds and whisk again to combine. For a smoother pudding, if desired, after the chia seeds have formed a gel, process using an immersion blender or blender until smooth. Cover and refrigerate overnight, or for at least 3 to 5 hours.

3. Serve chilled.

Ingredient Tip: Chia seeds are high in unsaturated fat. When the seed is exposed to water, the outer layer forms a gel that is not only high in soluble fiber but can also serve as a thickener for dishes such as puddings, oatmeal, and smoothies.

Per Serving: Calories: 183; Total Fat: 8g; Saturated Fat: 2g; Carbohydrates: 25g; Fiber: 8g; Sugar: 13g; Protein: 7g; Iron: 2mg; Sodium: 107mg

Baked Apple-Cranberry Compote

Prep time: 15 minutes / *Cook time:* 40 minutes

This compote leaves the house smelling divine and is a powerhouse of fall flavors. Enjoy alone or with vanilla ice cream, whipped cream, or even vanilla yogurt. To make this recipe oat-free, simply omit the oats and use ½ cup of crushed pecans.

2 tablespoons brown sugar

1 tablespoon vanilla extract

1 tablespoon ground cinnamon

1 teaspoon ground nutmeg

6 large apples, peeled, cored, and sliced

⅓ cup dried cranberries or ½ cup fresh cranberries

¼ cup water

½ cup rolled oats (optional)

SERVES 6

DAIRY-FREE
EGG-FREE
NUT-FREE
VEGAN

1. Preheat the oven to 350°F. Grease a large baking dish with oil or butter.

2. In a small bowl, mix the brown sugar, vanilla, cinnamon, and nutmeg. Place the apples and cranberries in the baking dish and pour the water over the top. Sprinkle the spice mixture over the top. Mix well to combine. Sprinkle the oats (if using) over the top.

3. Bake for 40 minutes, uncovered, until the apples are tender. Serve.

Per Serving: Calories: 155; Total Fat: 1g; Saturated Fat: 0g; Carbohydrates: 38g; Fiber: 6g; Sugar: 26g; Protein: 2g; Iron: 1mg; Sodium: 3mg

Ingredient Tip: There are over 2,500 types of apples grown in the United States (and 100 commercial varieties), but not all are suited for baking. Those with a softer flesh will turn to mush when baked and are better suited for applesauce (e.g., Macintosh). For an apple that holds it shape, choose Cortland, Fuji, Granny Smith, or Jonagold, to name a few.

Summer Berry Crisp

Prep time: 15 minutes / *Cook time:* 60 minutes

This bright crisp has a perfect streusel topping over bubbly summer fruits. It's an excellent way to use up extra fruit.

For the Topping

1 cup old-fashioned oats

½ cup chilled butter, cut into pieces

⅓ cup all-purpose, gluten-free flour

¼ cup light brown sugar

½ teaspoon salt

For the Berry Crisp

8 cups mixed chopped fresh or frozen summer fruit (peaches, cherries, plums, blueberries, and/or strawberries)

½ cup brown sugar

⅓ cup chia seeds

2 tablespoons freshly squeezed lemon juice

Pinch salt

SERVES 8

EGG-FREE

NUT-FREE

VEGETARIAN

Ingredient Tip: Using chia seeds instead of the traditional cornstarch adds a boost of fiber and omega-3 fatty acids to this dish.

Substitution Tip: To make this recipe oat-free, simply omit the oats and substitute with crushed pecans.

To Make the Topping

In a large bowl, combine the oats, butter, flour, brown sugar, and salt. Using your hands, mix and break apart the butter until the mixture is crumbly. Set aside.

To Make the Berry Crisp

1. Preheat the oven to 375°F.

2. In a bowl, toss together the fruit, brown sugar, chia seeds, lemon juice, and salt.

3. Transfer the fruit mixture to a 9-inch square baking dish. Sprinkle the oat topping over the top. Bake for about 1 hour, until the oats are crisp and brown.

4. Transfer to a wire rack and let cool before serving.

Per Serving: Calories: 304; Total Fat: 15g; Saturated Fat: 7g; Carbohydrates: 40g; Fiber: 8g; Sugar: 23g; Protein: 4g; Iron: 2mg; Sodium: 234mg

Chewy Chocolate Chip Bars

Prep time: 10 minutes / *Cook time:* 25 minutes

This recipe makes the perfect chewy chocolate chip blondie. If you prefer individual cookies, chill the dough for at least 4 hours prior to forming cookies.

2¼ cups all-purpose, gluten-free flour

½ teaspoon xanthan gum (if not already in the all-purpose flour)

1 teaspoon baking soda

1 teaspoon salt

1 cup packed brown sugar

¾ cup (1½ sticks) unsalted butter, melted

½ cup granulated sugar

2 large eggs

1½ teaspoons vanilla extract

1 cup semisweet chocolate chips

MAKES 20 BARS

NUT-FREE

VEGETARIAN

Prep Ahead Tip: For fresh-baked cookies anytime, combine the dough and form into logs. Wrap the dough in plastic wrap and freeze up to 1 month. When you're in the mood for cookies, cut off 2-inch sections and bake for 12 minutes.

1. Preheat the oven to 375°F. Line a 9-by-13-inch baking dish or rimmed baking sheet with parchment paper.

2. In a medium bowl, whisk together flour, xanthan gum (optional), baking soda, and salt. Set aside.

3. In a separate bowl, combine the brown sugar, butter, sugar, eggs, and vanilla. Mix well. Fold in the flour mixture and the chocolate chips and mix until combined. Pour the batter into the pan.

4. Bake for 25 minutes, until firm.

5. Allow to cool before cutting.

Per Serving (1 cookie): Calories: 189; Total Fat: 9g; Saturated Fat: 5g; Carbohydrates: 26g; Fiber: 2g; Sugar: 15g; Protein: 2g; Iron: 0mg; Sodium: 174mg

No-Bake Crustless Pumpkin Pie

Prep time: 5 minutes, plus 1 hour to chill

This recipe has all the flavor of pumpkin pie without any of the gluten, carbs, or effort. Simply combine and let sit for a few hours before enjoying pumpkin in all its glory.

1 cup pumpkin purée

1 (1-ounce) package instant vanilla pudding mix

½ cup whole milk

1 teaspoon pumpkin pie spice

1 cup whipped topping, divided

SERVES 4

NUT-FREE

VEGETARIAN

1. In large bowl, combine the pumpkin, pudding mix, milk, pumpkin pie spice, and ½ cup of the whipped topping.

2. Divide the pumpkin mixture between serving dishes. Spoon the remaining ½ cup whipped topping over the top of the cups.

3. Refrigerate for 1 to 2 hours before serving, until the filling has set. Serve with gluten-free graham crackers for crunch.

Substitution Tip: If you prefer an alternative to instant vanilla pudding, you can use ⅓ cup chia seeds, ⅓ cup maple syrup, and 1 teaspoon vanilla to help create the pudding consistency. For a smoother finish, blend before serving.

Per Serving: Calories: 158; Total Fat: 4g; Saturated Fat: 2g; Carbohydrates: 28g; Fiber: 2g; Sugar: 22g; Protein: 2g; Iron: 1mg; Sodium: 203mg

Chocolate-Drizzled Coconut Macaroons

Prep time: 10 minutes / *Cook time:* 25 minutes

This simple dessert creates the perfect cookie—soft and chewy on the inside with a rich chocolate shell.

1 (14-ounce) bag sweetened flaked coconut

¾ cup sweetened condensed milk

1 teaspoon vanilla extract

2 large egg whites

¼ teaspoon salt

4 ounces chopped semisweet chocolate

MAKES
20 MACAROONS

NUT-FREE

VEGETARIAN

Make Ahead Tip: These cookies stay very moist in a sealed container or bag for up to a week. They can also be frozen for up to 3 months.

Per Serving
(1 cookie): Calories: 139;
Total Fat: 9g;
Saturated Fat: 7g;
Carbohydrates: 13g;
Fiber: 2g; Sugar: 10g;
Protein: 2g; Iron: 3mg;
Sodium: 53mg

1. Preheat the oven to 325°F. Line two baking sheets with parchment paper.

2. In a medium bowl, mix together the coconut, condensed milk, and vanilla extract. Set aside.

3. In a separate bowl using a mixer on medium-high speed, beat the egg whites and salt until stiff peaks form, 6 to 8 minutes. Fold the egg whites into the coconut mixture.

4. Form small, 1-inch mounds of the mixture on the baking sheets, leaving space between each. Bake for 25 minutes. Remove from the oven and let cool completely.

5. Fill the bottom pot of a double boiler (or use a bowl sitting on top of a pan) one-third full of water and bring to a boil. Once boiling, reduce the heat to medium and place the chocolate in the metal bowl on top. Make sure the bottom of the bowl isn't touching the water. Stir the chocolate until melted, about 3 minutes. Avoid overheating it.

6. Drizzle the chocolate over the top of the cookies.

Raw Vegan Chocolate Cheesecake

Prep time: 15 minutes

No-bake cheesecakes are smooth as velvet and incredibly rich. Dairy won't be missed in this simple dessert.

For the Chocolate Crust

1½ cups almonds

2½ tablespoons maple syrup

2 tablespoons coconut oil or butter

2 tablespoons cocoa powder

½ teaspoon vanilla extract

Pinch salt

For the Chocolate Fudge Cheesecake

1 cup cashews

1 medium avocado

½ cup maple syrup

⅓ cup cocoa powder

¼ cup coconut oil or butter

1 teaspoon freshly squeezed lemon juice

1 tablespoon vanilla extract

Pinch salt

¼ cup slivered almonds (optional)

SERVES 8

30-MINUTE
DAIRY-FREE
EGG-FREE
VEGAN

Substitution Tip: If avocado is unavailable or you're looking for more nutrition, substitute 1 cup drained and rinsed chickpeas for the avocado.

To Make the Chocolate Crust

In a food processor, pulse the almonds, maple syrup, coconut oil, cocoa powder, and vanilla until it forms a crumble. Press into a parchment-lined 7-inch springform pan or pie pan. Set aside.

To Make the Chocolate Fudge Cheesecake

1. In a small bowl, soak the cashews for 15 minutes in very hot (but not boiling) water. Drain, rinse, and shake the cashews dry.

2. In a food processor, put in the cashews and blend about 2 minutes, until broken down. Add the avocado, maple syrup, cocoa powder, coconut oil, lemon juice, vanilla, and salt. Blend until smooth.

3. Pour the filling over crust and smooth with a spatula. Cover pan and refrigerate until firm.

4. Sprinkle the almonds (if using) over the top before serving for a little extra crunch and appearance.

Per Serving: Calories: 388; Total Fat: 28g; Saturated Fat: 10g; Carbohydrates: 31g; Fiber: 4g; Sugar: 20g; Protein: 7g; Iron: 2mg; Sodium: 7mg

Flourless Brownies

Prep time: 20 minutes / *Cook time:* 40 minutes

There's nothing more satisfying than a rich, chocolate brownie. Gluten-free brownies using alternative flours are often a bit dry and crumbly, but the black beans in this recipe provide all the gooey texture and rich chocolate flavor with none of the gluten. The beans disappear completely in this dish. Your guests will be scratching their heads trying to figure out the secret ingredient.

1 (15-ounce) can black beans, drained and rinsed or 1¾ cups cooked black beans

¾ cup cocoa powder

¼ cup maple syrup

3 tablespoons vegetable oil or melted butter

1 teaspoon vanilla extract

⅓ cup semisweet chocolate chips

2 large eggs or egg substitute

1½ teaspoons baking powder

1 teaspoon baking soda

¼ teaspoon salt

MAKES 16 BROWNIES

NUT-FREE

VEGETARIAN

Ingredient Tip: Using black beans instead of gluten-free flour in this recipe ensures a cake-like brownie that is also high in fiber, iron, and protein.

1. Preheat the oven to 350°F. Lightly grease an 8-inch square baking dish.

2. In a food processor or blender, combine the black beans, cocoa powder, maple syrup, vegetable oil, and vanilla and purée until smooth.

3. Pour the mixture into a mixing bowl. Fold in the chocolate chips, eggs, baking powder, baking soda, and salt until well combined. Pour the batter into the prepared baking pan.

4. Bake for 35 to 45 minutes, until the top is dry and the sides pull away from the pan.

5. Remove from the oven. Let cool before cutting and serving.

Per Serving: Calories: 120; Total Fat: 7g; Saturated Fat: 2g; Sodium: 101mg; Carbohydrates: 11g; Fiber: 2g; Sugar: 5g; Protein: 5g; Iron: 2mg

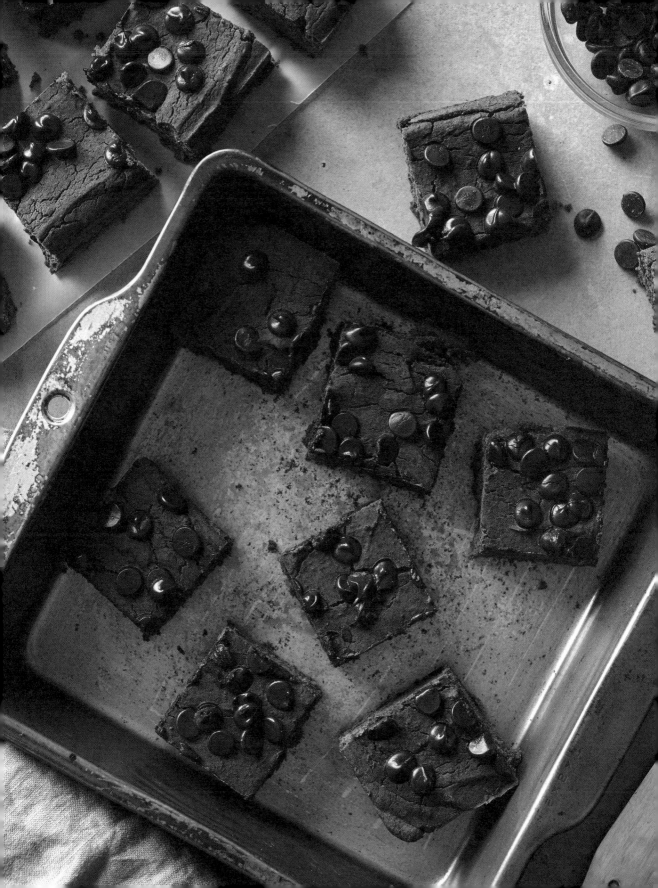

Master List of Foods to Avoid (and What to Substitute)

AVOID	SUBSTITUTION
Grains such as barley, bran, bulgur, durum, einkorn, emmer, farina, farro, kamut, rye	Rice, quinoa, millet, amaranth, and teff are great alternatives.
Pasta, noodles, couscous, orzo, udon	Potato, rice, quinoa, millet, and amaranth. Banza, Jovial, Barilla, and Trader Joe's have gluten-free options.
Wheat and any wheat flour	Use a premade flour blend, such as Bob's Red Mill or King Arthur. You can make your own by searching the internet for gluten-free flour blend recipes.
Bread, bagels, English muffins	Opt for gluten-free alternatives, such as Udi's, Rudi's, and Glutino. Try Canyon Bakehouse's Heritage-Style Whole-Wheat Bread, Schär's Hearty Grain, and Trader Joe's Gluten-Free Whole-Grain Bread.
Tortillas	Purchase a gluten-free variety such as Mission, Rudi's, BFree, Flatout, and Trader Joe's Brown Rice Tortilla wraps.
Soy sauce	Tamari, Bragg Liquid Aminos
Worcestershire sauce	Gluten-free variety (Lea and Perrins)
Crackers and matzo meal	Raw vegetables or rice crackers are great substitutes.

AVOID	SUBSTITUTION
Cookies	Purchase a gluten-free variety or make your own.
Cereal	Purchase a gluten-free brand.
Breaded products, including panko	Gluten-free breading Grilled (no breading) Baked (no breading)
Cream soups	Buy gluten-free or thicken your own with cornstarch or gluten-free flour.
Cream sauces and gravies	Make your own roux or gravy using a gluten-free flour.
Salad dressing	Use oil, vinegar, and/or lemon.
Veggie burgers	Make your own using beans and rice.
Meat substitutes made with wheat, such as seitan, chicken substitutes, sausage/bacon substitutes	Use tempeh, tofu, and/or beans for protein.
Oats	Purchase one labeled gluten-free to avoid cross contamination.
Malt, Malt vinegar	Red wine vinegar, white vinegar, balsamic vinegar
Wheat germ	Flaxseed
Wheat starch	Cornstarch can work as a thickening substitute. If the recipe relies on it for a chewy texture, there's no good substitute.

Resources

SUPPORT GROUPS

Organizations across the United States provide valuable support to those with celiac disease and advocate for the cause.

Beyond Celiac: www.beyondceliac.org

Celiac Disease Foundation: www.celiac.org

Gluten Intolerance Group: www.gluten.net

National Celiac Association: www.nationalceliac.org

WEBSITES

BeFreeForMe.com: Coupons and samples for gluten-free and food-allergy customers

Celiac.com: A helpful resource that covers numerous topics related to celiac disease

CeliacChicks.com: A blog and site promoting a hip and healthy gluten-free lifestyle

CeliacTravel.com: Gluten-free restaurant cards in many languages

DeletetheWheat.com: Nutrition counseling and consulting by Melinda Dennis, MS, RDN

GlutenFreeda.com: An online cooking magazine promoting healthy gluten-free recipes

GlutenFreeDietitian.com: Nutrition counseling and resources from Tricia Thompson, MS, RD

GlutenFreeDrugs.com: Lists of gluten-free drugs and definitions of common ingredients in over-the-counter and prescription drugs

GlutenFreeGirl.com: Blog and recipes

GlutenFreeGlobetrotter.com: Resources and blog about traveling while maintaining a gluten-free diet

GlutenFreeGoddess.Blogspot.com: Recipes and tips

GlutenFreeMD.com: Resources and information about celiac disease and gluten intolerance from Dr. Michelle Maria

GlutenFreeTravelSite.com: Resources and insights about eating gluten-free across the United States and abroad

GlutenFreeWatchdog.com: Reports and testing results on gluten-free products for consumers

JackieOurman.com: Celiac and allergy-friendly recipes

TheCeliacMD.com: Resources and recipes from Amy Burkhart, MD, RD

MAGAZINES

Allergic Living

Delight Gluten Free

Easy Eats

Gluten Free & More

Gluten-Free Living

Simply Gluten Free

APPS

AllergyEats: Guide to food allergy-friendly restaurants across the United States

Find Me Gluten Free: Reviews and guides to allergy-friendly restaurants across the United States

Fooducate Healthy Weight Loss & Calorie Counter: Scans and grades foods based on their ingredients. Learn nutrition basics and get recommendations for healthy alternatives.

Gluten Free Restaurant Cards: Over 40 card images in many languages to share with waitstaff and chefs to explain your dietary restrictions

Is It Gluten Free?: Provides verified gluten-free product information.

Sift Food Labels: Breaks down ingredient labels on products using the barcode on the package. Just scan the barcode and go!

The Gluten Free Scanner: Maintains a database of food and drink products within the United States to detect the presence of gluten. Find out immediately whether a product contains gluten by scanning its barcode with your phone's camera.

Index

Acknowledgments

Tremendous thank you to the Celiac Center at Beth Israel Deaconess Medical Center and Children's Hospital in Boston, Massachusetts, for welcoming me into the celiac community by supporting my graduate research. Additional thank you to the patients over the years at the Cambridge Health Alliance and beyond who have shown me that eating well is about more than food knowledge—it's about human connection. Finally (but most importantly), to my husband and children who not only support my passion and time spent in nutrition therapy but also my experiments in the kitchen.

About the Author

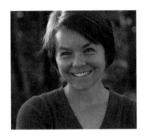

REBECCA TOUTANT, RD, LDN, CDE is a registered dietitian, personal trainer, and certified diabetes educator working in the suburbs of Boston, Massachusetts. Her background is as eclectic as her practice, working as a researcher, marketer, and counselor helping people of all ages navigate celiac disease, eating disorders, diabetes, and autism while leading full, nourishing lives. She began her career by exploring and publishing research with the experts at Beth Israel Deaconess Medical Center Celiac Center on the challenges young adults with celiac disease experience in their transition to college. She completed her undergraduate degree in Dietetics at the University of Wisconsin–Madison and her graduate degree in Health Communication at Emerson College and Tufts University School of Medicine. She can be found online at www.NourishingBitsandBites.com.